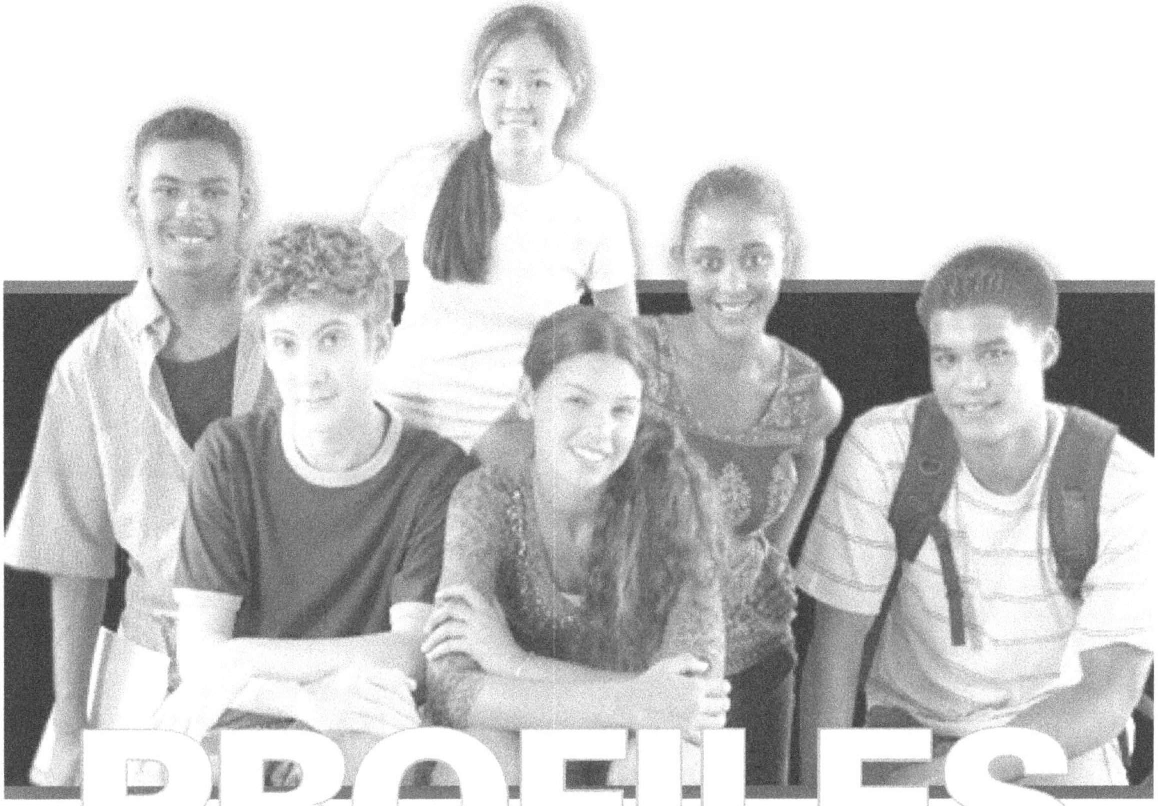

PROFILES 2006

School Health Profiles

Characteristics of Health Programs Among Secondary Schools

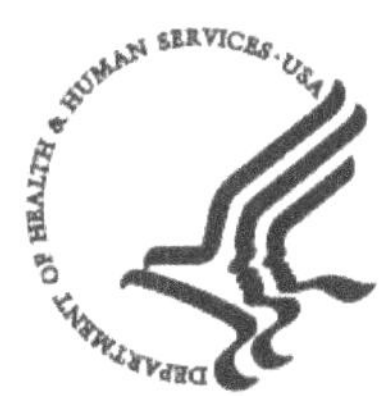

U.S. Department of Health and Human Services
Centers for Disease Control and Prevention
Coordinating Center for Health Promotion

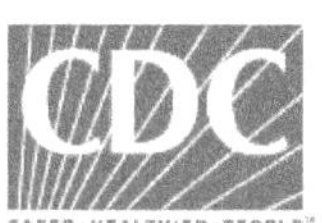

Suggested Citation

Balaji AB, Brener ND, McManus T, Hawkins J, Kann L, Speicher N. *School Health Profiles: Characteristics of Health Programs Among Secondary Schools 2006.* Atlanta: Centers for Disease Control and Prevention; 2008.

Ordering Information

For additional information about school health or to request free copies of this report, send an e-mail to Healthyyouth@cdc.gov, call 1-800-CDC-INFO (232-4636), or visit our Web site at http://www.cdc.gov/healthyyouth/profiles.

PROFILES 2006

School Health Profiles

Characteristics of Health Programs Among Secondary Schools

Alexandra B. Balaji, Ph.D.

Nancy D. Brener, Ph.D.

Tim McManus, M.S.

Joseph Hawkins, M.A.

Laura Kann, Ph.D.

Nancy Speicher, M.A.

U.S. DEPARTMENT OF HEALTH AND HUMAN SERVICES

CENTERS FOR DISEASE CONTROL AND PREVENTION

COORDINATING CENTER FOR HEALTH PROMOTION

TABLE OF CONTENTS

STATE AND LOCAL SCHOOL HEALTH PROFILES COORDINATORS v

INTRODUCTION 1

METHODOLOGY 3
- Sampling 3
- Data Collection 3
- Data Analysis 3

BACKGROUND 5
- Health Education 5
  - Requirements 5
  - Standards and Guidelines 5
  - Coordination of Health Education 6
  - Professional Preparation and Staff Development 6
- Physical Education 6
- Health Services 7
- Nutrition Services 8
- Healthy and Safe School Environment 8
  - Competitive Foods 8
  - Tobacco-Use Prevention 9
  - Violence Prevention 9
  - HIV Infection and AIDS Prevention 10
- Family and Community Involvement 10

RESULTS 11
- Health Education 11
  - Required Health Education 11
  - Materials Used in Required Health Education Courses 12
  - Content of Required Health Education Courses 13
    - Tobacco-Use Prevention Topics 14
    - Pregnancy, HIV, or STD Prevention Topics 16
    - Required HIV Prevention Units or Lessons 17
    - Nutrition and Dietary Behavior Topics 18
    - Physical Activity Topics 19

Teaching Methods in Required Health Education Courses....20
Coordination of Health Education....21
Professional Preparation and Staff Development....21
Physical Education and Physical Activity....26
Required Physical Education....26
Physical Activity....28
Nutrition Services....29
Healthy and Safe School Environment....29
Competitive Foods....29
Tobacco-Use Prevention....31
Violence Prevention....34
Health Services....35
Policies Related to HIV Infection and AIDS....36
Family and Community Involvement....37

TRENDS....39
Long-Term Trends....39
Short-Term Trends....41

DISCUSSION....43

REFERENCES....47

TABLES....54

STATE AND LOCAL SCHOOL HEALTH PROFILES COORDINATORS

Site	Coordinator	Affiliation
Alabama	Marchina Toodle, M.Ed.	Department of Education
Alaska	Todd Brocious	Department of Education & Early Development
Arizona	Catherine Osborn, M.Ed., M.P.A.	Department of Education
Arkansas	Kathleen Courtney, M.S.	Department of Education
Charlotte-Mecklenburg County, NC	Ruth Perez, Ed.D.	Charlotte-Mecklenburg Schools
Chicago, IL	Vicki Pittman, M.S., M.A.	Chicago Public Schools
Connecticut	Bonnie Edmondson, Ed.D.	Department of Education
Dallas, TX	Angelica Duran, L.M.S.W.	Dallas Independent School District
Delaware	Janet Ray, M.S.	Department of Education
District of Columbia	Marc Clark, Ph.D.	District of Columbia Public Schools
Florida	Antionette Meeks, Ed.D.	Department of Education
Georgia	Dafna Kanny, Ph.D.	Department of Human Resources
Hawaii	Dave Randall, M.Ed.	Department of Education
Hillsborough County, FL	Lloyd Zimet, M.P.H., Ph.D.	Hillsborough County Public Schools
Idaho	Patricia Stewart	Department of Education
Illinois	Glenn Steinhausen, Ph.D.	State Board of Education
Iowa	Sara Peterson, M.A.	Department of Education
Kansas	Allison Koonce, M.S.	Department of Health and Environment
Los Angeles, CA	Ric Loya, M.S.	Los Angeles Unified School District
Maine	Katherine Wilbur, M.Ed.	Department of Education
Massachusetts	Chiniqua Milligan, M.P.H.	Department of Education
Memphis, TN	Brenda McSparrin Gallagher, Ph.D.	Memphis City Schools
Miami, FL	Rodolfo Abella, Ph.D.	Miami-Dade County Public Schools
Michigan	Kim Kovalchick, M.S.W., M.P.H.	Department of Education
Mississippi	Stephanie Robinson, M.S.	Department of Education
Missouri	Kevin Miller, M.A.	Department of Elementary and Secondary Education
Montana	Susan Court	Office of Public Instruction
Nebraska	Julane Hill	Department of Education
New Hampshire	Mary Bubnis, M.Ed.	Department of Education
New York	Owen Donavan, M.S.E.	Department of Education
North Carolina	Sarah Langer, M.P.H.	Department of Public Instruction
North Dakota	Andrea Peña, M.A.	Department of Public Instruction
Orange County, FL	Kathleen Bowman, M.S.	Orange County Public Schools
Oregon	Nigel Chaumeton, Ph.D.	Department of Human Services
Pennsylvania	Shirley Black, M.Ed.	Department of Education
Philadelphia, PA	Bettyann Creighton, M.Ed.	School District of Philadelphia
Rhode Island	Jan Mermin, M.S.W.	Department of Elementary and Secondary Education
San Diego, CA	Marge Kleinsmith-Hildebrand, M.S.	San Diego Unified School District
San Francisco, CA	Phong Pham, M.A.	San Francisco Unified School District
South Carolina	Elaine Maney, M.P.H.	Department of Education
South Dakota	Karen Keyser	Department of Education
Tennessee	Jerry Swaim, M.S.	Department of Education
Texas	Marissa Rathbone, M.A.T.	Education Agency
Utah	Frank Wojtech, M.S.	Office of Education
Vermont	Karen Abbott	Department of Education
Virginia	Caroline Fuller, M.A.T.	Department of Education
Washington	Susan Richardson	Department of Health
West Virginia	Gus Nelson, M.S.	Department of Education

INTRODUCTION

In the United States, 54 million young people attend school for about six hours of class time approximately 180 days per year.[1] Schools are therefore in a unique position to help improve the health status of children and adolescents throughout the United States. In 1995, the Centers for Disease Control and Prevention (CDC), in collaboration with state and local education and health agencies, developed the School Health Profiles (Profiles) to measure health education practices and some school health policies. During the past 10 years, based on input from education and health agencies, Profiles has evolved to provide a more comprehensive assessment of school health policies and programs.

Profiles helps state and local education and health agencies monitor and assess characteristics of and trends in school health education; physical education; health services; school health policies related to human immunodeficiency virus (HIV) and acquired immunodeficiency syndrome (AIDS) prevention, tobacco-use prevention, violence prevention, physical activity, and competitive foods (foods and beverages sold outside of the U.S. Department of Agriculture [USDA] school meal programs); and family and community involvement in school health programs. Profiles has been conducted biennially since 1996 and includes state and local surveys of principals and lead health education teachers in middle and high schools.

The broad focus of Profiles provides some information on five of the eight components of a coordinated school health program (CSHP):[2]

- **Health education** provides students with a planned, sequential curriculum that addresses the physical, mental, emotional, and social dimensions of health. The curriculum is designed to motivate and assist students to maintain and improve their health, prevent disease, and reduce health-related risk behaviors. It allows students to develop and demonstrate increasingly sophisticated health-related knowledge, attitudes, skills, and practices.

- **Physical education** provides students with a planned, sequential curriculum that provides cognitive content and learning experiences in a variety of activity areas. Quality physical education should promote, through a variety of planned physical activities, each student's optimum physical, mental, emotional, and social development, and should promote activities and sports that all students enjoy and can pursue throughout their lives.

- **Health services** are provided for students to appraise, protect, and promote health. These services are designed to ensure access or referral to primary health care services or both, foster appropriate use of primary health care services, prevent and control communicable disease and other health problems, provide emergency care for illness or injury, promote and provide optimum sanitary conditions for a safe school facility and school environment, and provide educational and counseling opportunities for promoting and maintaining individual, family, and community health.

- **Healthy and safe school environment** refers to the physical and aesthetic surroundings and the psychosocial climate and culture of the school. Factors that influence the physical environment include the school building and the area surrounding it, any biological or chemical agents that are detrimental to health, and physical conditions such as temperature, noise, and lighting. The psychosocial environment includes the emotional and social conditions that affect the well-being of students and staff.

- **Family and community involvement** provides an integrated school, parent, and community approach for enhancing the health and well-being of students. School health advisory councils, coalitions, and broadly based constituencies for school health can build support for school health program efforts. Schools can actively solicit parent involvement and engage community resources and services to respond more effectively to the health-related needs of students.

This report summarizes 2006 Profiles data. For each middle or high school sampled, the principal and the lead health education teacher (the person who coordinates health education policies and programs within the school) each completed a self-administered questionnaire. Principal data from the 36 state and 12 local surveys with weighted data and lead health education teacher data from the 34 state and 12 local surveys with weighted data are included in this report.

Principal data from the remaining 8 state and 4 local surveys with unweighted data and lead health education teacher data from the remaining 10 state and 4 local surveys with unweighted data are not included in this report. One local survey with weighted data is not included in this report because permission to use the data was not granted to CDC. This report also examines both long-term (1996–2006) and short-term (2004–2006) trends in school health programs and policies.

METHODOLOGY

SAMPLING

Profiles employs random, systematic, equal-probability sampling strategies to produce representative samples of schools that serve students in grades 6 through 12 in each jurisdiction. In most states and cities, the sampling frame consists of all regular secondary public schools with one or more of grades 6 through 12. In 2006, 19 education and health agencies modified this procedure and invited all secondary schools, rather than just a sample, to participate.

DATA COLLECTION

The data are collected from each sampled school primarily during the spring semester, with the exception of Texas, which collected data during Fall 2006. Both the principal and lead health education teacher questionnaire booklets are mailed by the state or local education or health agency to the principal, who then designates the school's lead health education teacher to complete the teacher questionnaire.

Participation in the survey is confidential and voluntary; follow-up telephone calls and written reminders are used to encourage participation. The principal and teacher record their responses in the questionnaire booklets and return them directly to the state or local education or health agency.

DATA ANALYSIS

The data from states and cities that had response rates of 70% or greater and appropriate documentation (separately for the principal and teacher surveys) were weighted. The data are weighted to reflect the likelihood of principals or teachers being selected and to adjust for differing patterns of nonresponse.

This report represents information from the 34 states and 12 cities with weighted data from both principal and lead health education teacher surveys and 2 states with weighted data from the principal survey only (Table 1). Across states, the sample sizes of the principal surveys ranged from 68 to 661, and response rates ranged from 70% to 91%; across cities, the sample sizes ranged from 31 to 234, and response rates ranged from 71% to 98%. The sample sizes of the lead health education teacher surveys across states ranged from 68 to 659, and response rates ranged from 70% to 91%; across cities, the sample sizes ranged from 32 to 212, and the response rates ranged from 70% to 100%. SAS software was used to compute point estimates.[3] Medians and ranges are presented separately for states and cities.

The Wilcoxon rank-sum test was used to test for differences between 1996 and 2006 data and between 2004 and 2006 data across states and cities.[4] This is a nonparametric analogue to a two sample t-test. This statistical procedure rank-ordered all sites for both years separately for states and cities, summed the ranks separately by year and for states and cities, and compared the rank sums separately for states and cities to determine whether the distribution of a variable was the same for 1996 and 2006, or for 2004 and 2006.

Assuming the percentages have an underlying continuous distribution, the distribution of ranks is approximately normal; however, because of the small sample sizes, p values were obtained from the t distribution rather than the normal distribution. Because multiple comparisons were made, the distributions were considered statistically significantly different if p was less than 0.01.

To analyze long-term trends and short-term trends, many variables from the 1996 and 2004 Profiles were recalculated so that the denominators used for each year of data were defined identically. In most cases, this denominator included all schools, rather than a subset of schools. As a result of this recalculation, percentages previously reported for the 1996 or 2004 Profiles might differ from those reported here. Only estimates based on the same denominator should be compared.

BACKGROUND

HEALTH EDUCATION

Requirements

Health education curricula should be planned, sequential, and implemented for all grades in elementary and middle schools and through at least one semester in high schools.[5,6] Health education should address the physical, mental, emotional, and social dimensions of health and be age appropriate.[7] School health education provides students with the knowledge, attitudes, and skills they need to avoid or modify behaviors related to the leading causes of death, illness, and injury during youth and adulthood.

A comprehensive health education curriculum includes a variety of topics, such as personal health, family health, community health, consumer health, environmental health, sexuality education, mental and emotional health, injury prevention and safety, nutrition, prevention and control of disease, and substance use and abuse.

Standards and Guidelines

The *National Health Education Standards: Achieving Health Literacy* provides a framework for designing or selecting health education curricula and allocating instructional resources, as well as providing a basis for the assessment of student achievement. The *National Health Education Standards* also offers students, families, and communities concrete expectations for health education. The Joint Committee on National Health Education Standards released the first set of standards in 1995.[8] The National Health Education Standards Review and Revision Panel released the following updated set of eight standards in 2007:[9]

1. Students will comprehend concepts related to health promotion and disease prevention to enhance health.

2. Students will analyze the influence of family, peers, culture, media, technology, and other factors on health behaviors.

3. Students will demonstrate the ability to access valid information and products and services to enhance health.

4. Students will demonstrate the ability to use interpersonal communication skills to enhance health and avoid or reduce health risks.

5. Students will demonstrate the ability to use decision-making skills to enhance health.

6. Students will demonstrate the ability to use goal-setting skills to enhance health.

7. Students will demonstrate the ability to practice health-enhancing behaviors and avoid or reduce health risks.

8. Students will demonstrate the ability to advocate for personal, family, and community health.

School health education is supported by the U.S. Department of Health and Human Services' *Healthy People 2010*,[10] Objective 7-2: "Increase the proportion of middle, junior high, and senior high schools that provide school health education to prevent health problems in the following areas: unintentional injury; violence; suicide; tobacco use and addiction; alcohol and other drug use; unintended pregnancy, HIV/AIDS, and STD (sexually transmitted disease) infection; unhealthy dietary patterns; inadequate physical activity; and environmental health."

Coordination of Health Education

A necessary component of effective health education is management and coordination by a professional who is trained in health education.[11] That person may work at either the school or the school district level. Curriculum planning and development is enhanced when schools have a school health coordinator. Collaboration between health education teachers and other school staff members also improves the implementation of health education curricula. To supplement a separate health education course, health-related information can be included in a range of disciplines, including physical education, the sciences, mathematics, language arts, social studies, home economics, and the arts.[12]

Professional Preparation and Staff Development

The quality of school health education is determined, in part, by teacher preparation.[7] Professional development for teachers through continuing education and training is critical for the implementation of effective school health education.[13-15] Professional development for health education teachers should focus on strategies that actively engage students and help students master important health information and skills.[7] Studies have shown that teachers who receive training tend to implement health education with more fidelity than do teachers who do not receive such training, resulting in increased knowledge gain among students.[16]

PHYSICAL EDUCATION

Regular physical activity can reduce risk for the development of chronic diseases among adults,[17] including cardiovascular disease,[18] cancer,[19] and diabetes.[20] Because participation in physical activity as a young person influences participation in physical activity as an adult, it can contribute to decreased risk for the development of such chronic diseases.[21] Regular participation in physical activity as a young person contributes to healthy bone and muscle development, reduces feelings of depression and anxiety, and promotes psychological well-being.[21] Further, regular physical activity reduces risk for the development of overweight among youth. In 2004, 18.8% of 6-year-olds to 11-year-olds and 17.4% of 12-year-olds to 19-year-olds were considered obese, and an additional 20.4% of 6-year-olds to 11-year-olds and 15.3% of 12-year-olds to 19-year-olds were considered overweight.[*,22] Many youth become less active as they move from childhood into adolescence and adulthood.[23-26]

Schools can play an important role in providing opportunities for physical activity, and instructing students on ways to be physically active and the benefits of physical activity. CDC's *Guidelines for School and Community Programs to Promote Lifelong Physical Activity among Young People*[27] recommends that schools adopt a comprehensive approach to physical activity by requiring daily physical education, teaching skills and knowledge for maintaining and enjoying a physically active lifestyle, and providing extracurricular physical activity programs. In 2002, the Task Force on Community Preventive Services published recommendations that communities can implement to increase physical activity among young people. The task force strongly recommended modifying school-based physical education curricula and policies to increase the amount of time students spend in moderate to vigorous activity while in physical education classes.[28] Increasing the amount of time students are active can be achieved either by increasing the amount of time spent in physical education class or by increasing the amount of time students are active during already scheduled physical education classes.

* Note that these classifications of obese and overweight do not reflect the classifications used in the article cited but rather the June 2007 recommendations from the Expert Committee on the Assessment, Prevention, and Treatment of Child and Adolescent Overweight and Obesity convened by the American Medical Association (AMA) and cofunded by AMA in collaboration with the Health Resources and Services Administration and the CDC.

To support quality physical education, The National Association for Sport and Physical Education published the second edition of the *National Standards for Physical Education* in 2004.[29] The importance of physical education and activity in promoting the health of young people is also supported by the following *Healthy People 2010*[10] objectives:

- **22-6.** Increase the proportion of adolescents who engage in moderate physical activity for at least 30 minutes on 5 or more of the previous 7 days.
- **22-7.** Increase the proportion of adolescents who engage in vigorous physical activity that promotes cardiorespiratory fitness 3 or more days per week for 20 or more minutes per occasion.
- **22-8.** Increase the proportion of the nation's public and private schools that require daily physical education for all students.
- **22-9.** Increase the proportion of adolescents who participate in daily school physical education.
- **22-10.** Increase the proportion of adolescents who spend at least 50% of school physical education class time being physically active.
- **22-12.** Increase the proportion of the nation's public and private schools that provide access to their physical activity spaces and facilities for all persons outside of normal school hours.

HEALTH SERVICES

According to the American Academy of Pediatrics (AAP), at a minimum, schools should provide the following three types of services: 1) state-mandated services, including health screenings, verification of immunization status, and infectious disease reporting, 2) assessment of minor health complaints, medication administration, and care for students with special health care needs, and 3) capability to handle emergencies and other urgent situations.[30] More comprehensive services might include administration of immunizations, case management, wellness promotion, and patient education, as well as services for students with special needs, such as physical therapy.

School nurses play many roles, but their main purpose is to support student success by providing health care assessment, intervention, and follow-up for all children within the school setting.[31] The importance of having sufficient school nurses for all students is reflected in *Healthy People 2010*[10] Objective 7-4, "to increase the proportion of the nation's elementary, middle, and high schools that have a nurse-to-student ratio of at least 1 to 750."

Asthma is a chronic illness that has increased in prevalence since 1980.[32] The impact of illness and death due to asthma is disproportionately higher among low-income populations, racial and ethnic minorities, boys, and children in inner cities.[32-34] In 2005, 142.2 per 1,000 children ages 5–17 had a diagnosis of asthma in their lifetime.[35] In 2002, children made five million visits to doctors' offices and hospital outpatient departments, 727,000 visits to hospital emergency departments, and had 196,000 hospitalizations due to asthma. An estimated 14.7 million lost school days are attributed to asthma among school-aged children.[33]

Although asthma cannot be cured, it can be controlled with proper diagnosis and appropriate care and management activities. Schools can help students manage their asthma by adopting policies and procedures to create safe and supportive learning environments for students with asthma. In *Strategies for Addressing Asthma Within a Coordinated School Health Program*,[36] CDC recommends obtaining a written action plan for all students with asthma and ensuring that students have immediate access to medications, including allowing students to carry and self-administer medications. *Healthy People 2010*[10] identifies the following objectives to effectively manage and improve the quality of life of persons with asthma:

- **24-4.** Reduce activity limitations among persons with asthma.
- **24-5.** Reduce the number of school or work days missed by persons with asthma due to asthma.

NUTRITION SERVICES

The need to promote healthy eating among youth has intensified as a result of the growing national epidemic of obesity.[22] Healthy eating is also important in the prevention of type 2 diabetes, the prevalence of which has increased dramatically among young people; type 2 diabetes also is often associated with obesity.[37,38] Schools are in a unique position to promote healthy dietary behaviors and to help ensure appropriate nutrient intake. In 2004, more than half (54%) of school-aged children in the United States received either school breakfast or school lunch, and 1 in 6 received both.[39] School nutrition services staff can promote healthy eating through the foods they make available each day in the school cafeteria and the opportunities they have to reinforce nutrition education taught in the classroom.

The goal of school nutrition services is to provide nutritionally appropriate meals that are accessible to all students at a reasonable price in a pleasant and comfortable environment.[5] School meal programs should offer a variety of foods that adhere to the recommendations of the Dietary Guidelines for Americans, including offering fresh fruit, vegetables, and whole grain products. School menus should reflect the ethnic and cultural food preferences of students, including those with special dietary requirements, and encourage student and family involvement in menu planning and taste testing.

HEALTHY AND SAFE SCHOOL ENVIRONMENT

Competitive Foods

USDA defines competitive foods as those foods and beverages sold at school outside of the USDA school meal program, regardless of their nutritional value.[40] The only federal regulation on sale of foods and beverages outside of the school meal program addresses foods of minimal nutritional value (FMNV).[†, 41] Currently, federal regulations require only that a school prohibit access to FMNV in food service areas during mealtimes. The average young person consumes more than 10% of calories from saturated fat, less than two thirds of the recommended intake of calcium, and more than double the recommended amount of sodium.[42-44] For both boys and girls aged 9 to 13 years, 21% derive more than one quarter of their energy intake from added sugars.[45]

Schools have a unique opportunity to provide students with healthy dietary choices and to help students learn about healthy food choices. The Child Nutrition and WIC Reauthorization Act of 2004 requires school districts that participate in the USDA National School Lunch Program or School Breakfast Program to develop a local wellness policy that must address nutrition education and provide nutrition guidelines for all foods available on school campuses.[46] The recently released Institute of Medicine report, *Nutrition Standards for Foods in Schools: Leading the Way Toward Healthier Youth*[47] provides specific recommendations for foods and beverages sold outside of the school meal programs that schools, districts, and states should consider when developing or strengthening policies related to nutrition in schools.

† Foods of minimal nutritional value (FMNV) are defined as items that provide less than 5% of the U.S. recommended daily allowance per serving for each of eight essential nutrients. FMNV include carbonated soft drinks, water ices, chewing gum, and certain candies made largely from sweeteners, such as hard candy and jelly beans. Under the federal regulations, foods such as potato chips, chocolate bars, and doughnuts are not considered FMNV and can be sold in the cafeteria or elsewhere in the school at any time.

The implementation of these recommendations, the USDA local wellness policy, and other initiatives helps support the achievement of the *Healthy People 2010*[10] Objective 19-15: to increase the proportion of children and adolescents aged 6 to 19 years whose intake of meals and snacks at school contributes to good overall dietary quality.

Tobacco-Use Prevention

Tobacco use is the single leading preventable cause of death in the United States. During 1997–2001, smoking resulted in an estimated annual average of 259,494 deaths among men and 178,408 deaths among women in the United States.[48] Approximately 82% of adults who ever smoked daily tried their first cigarette before age 18 years.[49] Thus, to be most effective, school-based programs must target young people before they initiate tobacco use or drop out of school. CDC's *Guidelines for School Health Programs to Prevent Tobacco Use and Addiction*[50] recommend strategies to aid schools in preventing tobacco use among youth. The following are key elements of those strategies:

- Develop and enforce a school policy on tobacco use that prohibits tobacco use by students, school staff, parents, and visitors on school property, in school buildings, in all school vehicles, and at school functions away from school property.

- Prohibit tobacco advertising in school buildings, on school property, and in school publications.

- Provide instruction about the negative consequences of short-term and long-term tobacco use, social influences on tobacco use, peer norms regarding tobacco use, and refusal skills.

- Provide tobacco-use prevention education for students in kindergarten through grade 12.

- Provide program-specific training for teachers.

- Support cessation efforts among students and staff who use tobacco.

To be comprehensive, a tobacco-use prevention policy should prohibit all tobacco use by students, faculty, staff, and visitors during school and nonschool hours; in school buildings; on school grounds; in school buses or other vehicles used to transport students; and at off-campus, school-sponsored events.[50] Instituting such a policy can assist schools in achieving *Healthy People 2010*[10] Objective 27-11: to increase tobacco-free environments in schools, including all school facilities, property, vehicles, and events.

Violence Prevention

In 2003, unintentional injuries, suicide, and homicide accounted for 48.5% of all deaths among children aged 10 to 14 years and 74.9% of all deaths among adolescents aged 15 to 19 years.[51] The No Child Left Behind Act of 2001 authorizes federal funds for school programs to prevent violence in and around schools.[52] CDC's *School Health Guidelines to Prevent Unintentional Injury and Violence*[53] identifies the following strategies for school health efforts to prevent unintentional injury, violence, and suicide:

- Establish social and physical environments that promote safety and prevent unintentional injuries, violence, and suicide.

- Implement health and safety education to help students adopt and maintain safe lifestyles.

- Establish mechanisms for short-term and long-term response to crises, disasters, and injuries.

Healthy People 2010[10] Objective 15-39 calls for the reduction of weapon carrying by adolescents on school property.

HIV Infection and AIDS Prevention

Advances in drug therapies have extended the lives of people living with HIV infection and AIDS. Children are living longer with the disease and thus have a direct impact upon schools as they enter the school system. In 2005, 1,255 young people aged 13 to 19 years were diagnosed with HIV/AIDS, for a cumulative total (through 2005) of 5,311 HIV/AIDS cases in this age group.[54] Consistent condom use and HIV testing are important strategies for preventing the transmission of HIV. Nationwide, 62.8% of currently sexually active students in grades 9 through 12 had used a condom during last sexual intercourse while only 11.9% of students in grades 9 through 12 had been tested for HIV.[55]

School health policies that address issues raised by HIV infection and AIDS are critical for protecting the rights of affected students and school staff members. The National Association of State Boards of Education provides policy recommendations to guide educators in addressing these issues,[56] including:

- The right to school attendance for students with HIV infection or AIDS.
- Nondiscrimination for employees with HIV infection or AIDS.
- The right to privacy regarding HIV infection status.
- Adherence to infection-control guidelines.
- Accommodations for students living with HIV infection or AIDS to facilitate their participation in school-sponsored physical activities.
- An HIV infection prevention education program.
- Confidential counseling for students.
- A planned HIV education program for staff.
- Provisions for school administrators to notify students, parents, and school personnel about current policies concerning HIV infection and AIDS.

FAMILY AND COMMUNITY INVOLVEMENT

Partnerships between schools, families, and community members are key elements of effective school health programs.[57] Schools that have a good relationship with families and community members are more likely to gain their cooperation with school health efforts. These relationships also increase the probability of successful school health programs and improved student health outcomes.[58,59] Interventions aimed at preventing and treating childhood obesity,[60] school-based tobacco-use prevention programs,[61] and asthma interventions[62,63] have all been found to be more effective when they involve parents and community organizations. Family and community involvement is especially important when addressing topics that can be emotionally charged, such as the prevention of HIV, other STDs, and pregnancy.[64] Without parental support of HIV, other STD, and pregnancy prevention education programs and policies, they cannot be sustained.[65,66]

RESULTS

HEALTH EDUCATION

Required Health Education

Required health education is defined on the Profiles questionnaire as instruction about health topics that students must receive for graduation or promotion from school. Many schools require health education for students in grades 6 through 12. The percentage of all schools that required health education for students in any of grades 6 through 12 ranged from 55.6% to 99.4% (median: 91.5%) across states and from 56.0% to 100.0% (median: 87.2%) across cities (Table 2).

A required health education course is taught as a separate semester-long, quarter-long, or year-long unit of instruction for which the student receives credit. The percentage of all schools that required students to take only one required health education course ranged from 12.5% to 82.4% across states (median: 39.4%) and from 0.0% to 74.7% across cities (median: 44.5%) (Table 2). The percentage of all schools that required students to take two or more required health education courses ranged from 8.1% to 79.3% across states (median: 43.0%) and from 0.0% to 66.9% across cities (median: 16.1%).

Among schools that required health education for students in any of grades 6 through 12, schools taught required health education in the following ways:

- The percentage of schools that taught required health education in a combined health education and physical education course ranged from 32.8% to 98.0% across states (median: 63.1%) and from 12.4% to 100.0% across cities (median: 68.4%) (Table 2).
- The percentage of schools that taught required health education in a course mainly about another subject other than health education, such as science, social studies, home economics, or English, ranged from 7.2% to 37.4% across states (median: 19.6%) and from 0.0% to 90.9% across cities (median: 38.9%) (Table 2).

Among schools that required a health education course for students in any of grade 6 through grade 12, some schools required that students who fail the course repeat it. The percentage of these schools that required students to repeat a required health education course ranged from 35.0% to 95.4% (median: 55.4%) across states and from 35.1% to 86.2% (median: 60.2%) across cities (Table 2).

Among schools with students in particular grades, the percentage of schools across states that taught a required health education course in that grade ranged from 11.8% to 93.2% (median: 51.3%) in grade 6, 11.4% to 93.3% (median: 62.5%) in grade 7, 15.0% to 93.3% (median: 61.1%) in grade 8, 7.9% to 86.1% (median: 54.8%) in grade 9, 9.0% to 83.9% (median: 40.8%) in grade 10, 1.9% to 77.2% (median: 16.7%) in grade 11, and from 1.9% to 73.7% (median: 14.7%) in grade 12 (Table 3, Figure 1).

Among schools with students in particular grades, the percentage of schools across cities that taught a required health education course in that grade ranged from 0.0% to 100.0% (median: 37.1%) in grade 6, 0.0% to 100.0% (median: 37.0%) in grade 7, 0.0% to 100.0% (median: 25.1%) in grade 8, 0.0% to 100.0% (median: 36.4%) in grade 9, 0.0% to 58.8% (median: 22.9%) in grade 10, 0.0% to 42.3% (median: 11.3%) in grade 11, and from 0.0% to 37.3% (median: 10.2%) in grade 12 (Table 3, Figure 1).

FIGURE 1. Median percentage of schools that taught a required health education course in each grade,* School Health Profiles, 2006.

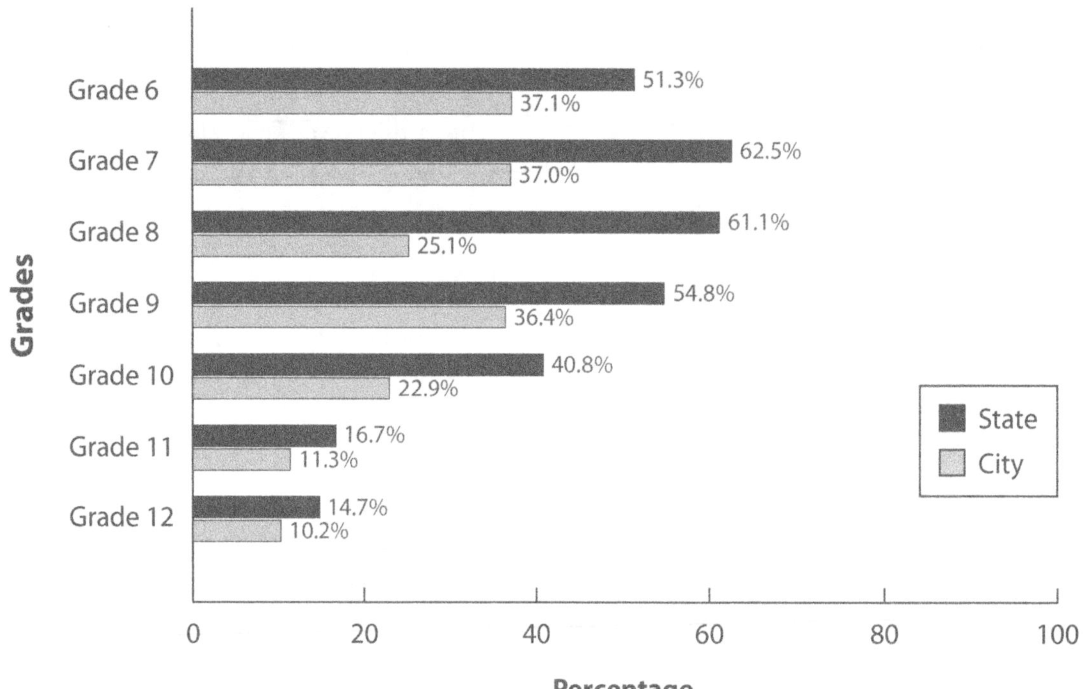

* Among schools with students in each grade.

Materials Used in Required Health Education Courses

Many schools required that teachers use specific materials in a required health education course. The percentage of all schools that required use of specific materials‡ ranged as follows (Table 4):

- **The National Health Education Standards:** from 24.7% to 76.9% across states (median: 44.1%) and from 0.0% to 63.7% across cities (median: 33.3%).
- **Any state-developed, district-developed, or school-developed curriculum:** from 36.3% to 95.9% (median: 75.3%) across states and from 0.0% to 97.1% across cities (median: 48.9%).
- **A commercially developed curriculum:** from 15.0% to 43.9% across states (median: 22.9%) and from 0.0% to 58.4% across cities (median: 20.6%).
- **A commercially developed student textbook:** from 17.6% to 80.7% across states (median: 43.9%) and from 0.0% to 83.9% across cities (median: 32.7%).
- **A commercially developed teacher's guide:** from 15.8% to 71.0% across states (median: 37.1%) and from 0.0% to 67.3% across cities (median: 34.8%).
- **Health education performance assessment materials:** from 23.0% to 70.5% across states (median: 36.3%) and from 0.0% to 59.2% across cities (median: 26.7%).

‡ Schools could report use of one or more types of material.

- **Materials from health organizations** such as the American Heart Association or the American Cancer Society: from 14.5% to 45.6% across states (median: 30.3%) and from 0.0% to 55.1% across cities (median: 30.7%).

Content of Required Health Education Courses

Required health education courses aim to increase student knowledge about a variety of health-related topics. The percentage of all schools that tried to increase student knowledge on specific health-related topics in a required health education course during the 2005–2006 school year ranged as follows (Tables 5a, b, c):

- **Alcohol-use or other drug-use prevention:** from 43.9% to 99.0% across states (median: 86.8%) and from 0.0% to 100.0% across cities (median: 57.6%).

- **Asthma awareness:** from 25.3% to 71.6% across states (median: 48.3%) and from 0.0% to 76.8% across cities (median: 36.9%).

- **Consumer health, such as choosing sources of health-related information, products, and services wisely:** from 34.8% to 95.5% across states (median: 77.4%) and from 0.0% to 95.0% across cities (median: 52.1%).

- **Cardiopulmonary resuscitation (CPR):** from 23.6% to 78.6% across states (median: 53.4%) and from 0.0% to 68.3% across cities (median: 46.6%).

- **Dental and oral health:** from 34.1% to 87.4% across states (median: 55.2%) and from 0.0% to 91.7% across cities (median: 41.3%).

- **Emotional and mental health:** from 40.9% to 98.4% across states (median: 83.1%) and from 0.0% to 98.9% across cities (median: 57.2%).

- **Environmental health, such as how air and water quality can affect health:** from 33.5% to 83.2% across states (median: 59.9%) and from 0.0% to 84.8% across cities (median: 47.2%).

- **First aid:** from 28.6% to 88.2% across states (median: 61.9%) and from 0.0% to 80.8% across cities (median: 47.9%).

- **Foodborne illness prevention:** from 29.2% to 84.5% across states (median: 61.4%) and from 0.0% to 88.9% across cities (median: 45.3%).

- **Growth and development:** from 40.3% to 96.5% across states (median: 80.6%) and from 0.0% to 98.7% across cities (median: 54.2%).

- **HIV prevention:** from 35.6% to 99.3% across states (median: 84.2%) and from 0.0% to 100.0% across cities (median: 57.2%).

- **Human sexuality:** from 28.9% to 96.9% across states (median: 76.3%) and from 0.0% to 97.3% across cities (median: 56.2%).

- **Immunizations:** from 24.1% to 79.4% across states (median: 51.0%) and from 0.0% to 78.7% across cities (median: 37.3%).

- **Injury prevention and safety:** from 35.0% to 93.9% across states (median: 77.6%) and from 0.0% to 88.7% across cities (median: 52.3%).

- **Nutrition and dietary behavior:** from 43.1% to 98.6% across states (median: 85.8%) and from 0.0% to 100.0% across cities (median: 57.2%).

- **Physical activity and fitness:** from 44.0% to 98.9% across states (median: 86.5%) and from 0.0% to 100.0% across cities (median: 56.3%).

- **Pregnancy prevention:** from 29.6% to 99.3% across states (median: 80.0%) and from 0.0% to 100.0% across cities (median: 56.2%).
- **STD prevention:** from 30.8% to 98.9% across states (median: 79.9%) and from 0.0% to 100.0% across cities (median: 57.2%).
- **Suicide prevention:** from 32.6% to 89.5% across states (median: 66.0%) and from 0.0% to 91.9% across cities (median: 49.3%).
- **Sun safety or skin cancer prevention:** from 37.3% to 85.7% across states (median: 65.9%) and from 0.0% to 87.9% across cities (median: 43.3%).
- **Tobacco-use prevention:** from 42.9% to 99.0% across states (median: 86.6%) and from 0.0% to 100.0% across cities (median: 57.2%).
- **Violence prevention, such as bullying, fighting, or homicide:** from 39.7% to 95.3% across states (median: 78.7%) and from 0.0% to 95.2% across cities (median: 57.2%).

Required health education courses also aim to improve student skills for adopting, practicing, and maintaining healthy behaviors. The percentage of all schools that tried to improve specific student skills in a required health education course during the 2005–2006 school year ranged as follows (Table 6):

- **Finding valid information or services related to personal health and wellness:** from 35.7% to 96.7% across states (median: 79.2%) and from 0.0% to 97.2% across cities (median: 54.4%).
- **Influence of media on personal health and wellness:** from 37.6% to 96.7% across states (median: 80.6%) and from 0.0% to 97.5% across cities (median: 54.4%).
- **Communication skills, such as how to ask for assistance with a health-related problem:** from 36.8% to 94.1% across states (median: 77.2%) and from 0.0% to 100.0% across cities (median: 54.4%).
- **Decision-making skills, such as deciding to get appropriate health screenings and exams:** from 34.6% to 94.9% across states (median: 77.9%) and from 0.0% to 92.1% across cities (median: 57.2%).
- **Goal-setting skills, such as setting a goal for improving personal health habits:** from 40.3% to 98.0% across states (median: 81.5%) and from 0.0% to 97.4% across cities (median: 54.4%).
- **Conflict resolution skills, such as techniques to resolve interpersonal conflicts without fighting:** from 39.1% to 95.6% across states (median: 79.7%) and from 0.0% to 94.5% across cities (median: 57.2%).
- **Resisting peer pressure to engage in unhealthy behavior related to personal health and wellness:** from 42.0% to 98.8% across states (median: 86.0%) and from 0.0% to 100.0% across cities (median: 55.4%).

Tobacco-Use Prevention Topics

Tobacco-use prevention topics taught in a required health education course included health outcomes and risks of tobacco use, external influences on tobacco use, and skills to avoid and to stop using tobacco. The percentage of all schools that taught about health outcomes and risks of tobacco use in a required health education course during the 2005–2006 school year ranged as follows (Table 7a):

- **Addictive effects of nicotine in tobacco products:** from 40.8% to 99.0% across states (median: 85.6%) and from 0.0% to 100.0% across cities (median: 56.8%).

- **Benefits of not smoking cigarettes (including long-term and short-term health benefits, social benefits, environmental benefits, and financial benefits):** from 42.0% to 98.7% across states (median: 85.9%) and from 0.0% to 100.0% across cities (median: 56.8%).

- **Benefits of not using smokeless tobacco:** from 37.6% to 98.3% across states (median: 81.4%) and from 0.0% to 98.7% across cities (median: 49.3%).

- **Short-term and long-term health consequences of cigarette smoking (such as stained teeth, bad breath, heart disease, and cancer):** from 41.3% to 99.0% across states (median: 86.2%) and from 0.0% to 100.0% across cities (median: 56.8%).

- **Short-term and long-term health consequences of using smokeless tobacco:** from 38.5% to 98.3% across states (median: 83.3%) and from 0.0% to 97.5% across cities (median: 53.9%).

- **Health effects of environmental tobacco smoke (ETS) or second-hand smoke:** from 40.2% to 98.3% across states (median: 84.2%) and from 0.0% to 98.9% across cities (median: 54.5%).

- **Short-term and long-term risks of cigar smoking:** from 35.9% to 91.0% across states (median: 71.7%) and from 0.0% to 93.9% across cities (median: 48.9%).

The percentage of all schools that taught about external influences on tobacco use in a required health education course during the 2005–2006 school year ranged as follows (Table 7b):

- **Influence of families on tobacco use:** from 35.7% to 97.1% across states (median: 82.2%) and from 0.0% to 97.6% across cities (median: 53.2%).

- **Influence of the media on tobacco use:** from 38.1% to 98.7% across states (median: 83.9%) and from 0.0% to 100.0% across cities (median: 56.8%).

- **Social or cultural influences on tobacco use:** from 36.5% to 95.0% across states (median: 78.8%) and from 0.0% to 96.3% across cities (median: 56.8%).

- **How many young people use tobacco:** from 37.2% to 96.6% across states (median: 80.1%) and from 0.0% to 96.6% across cities (median: 55.7%).

The percentage of all schools that taught skills to avoid and to stop using tobacco in a required health education course during the 2005–2006 school year ranged as follows (Table 7c):

- **Resisting peer pressure to use tobacco:** from 40.0% to 97.9% across states (median: 83.7%) and from 0.0% to 98.9% across cities (median: 56.8%).

- **Making a personal commitment not to use tobacco:** from 32.2% to 84.5% across states (median: 64.1%) and from 0.0% to 86.9% across cities (median: 49.0%).

- **How students can influence or support others to prevent tobacco use:** from 36.7% to 96.8% across states (median: 77.8%) and from 0.0% to 97.7% across cities (median: 54.7%).

- **How to find valid information or services related to tobacco-use prevention or cessation:** from 33.1% to 93.2% across states (median: 69.3%) and from 0.0% to 92.7% across cities (median: 50.0%).

- **How students can influence or support others in efforts to quit using tobacco:** from 35.5% to 95.1% across states (median: 75.3%) and from 0.0% to 95.3% across cities (median: 54.7%).

FIGURE 2. Median percentage of all schools that taught all 16 tobacco-use prevention topics; all 11 pregnancy, HIV,* or STD† prevention topics; all 14 nutrition and dietary behavior topics; or all 13 physical activity topics in a required health education course during the 2005–2006 school year, School Health Profiles, 2006.

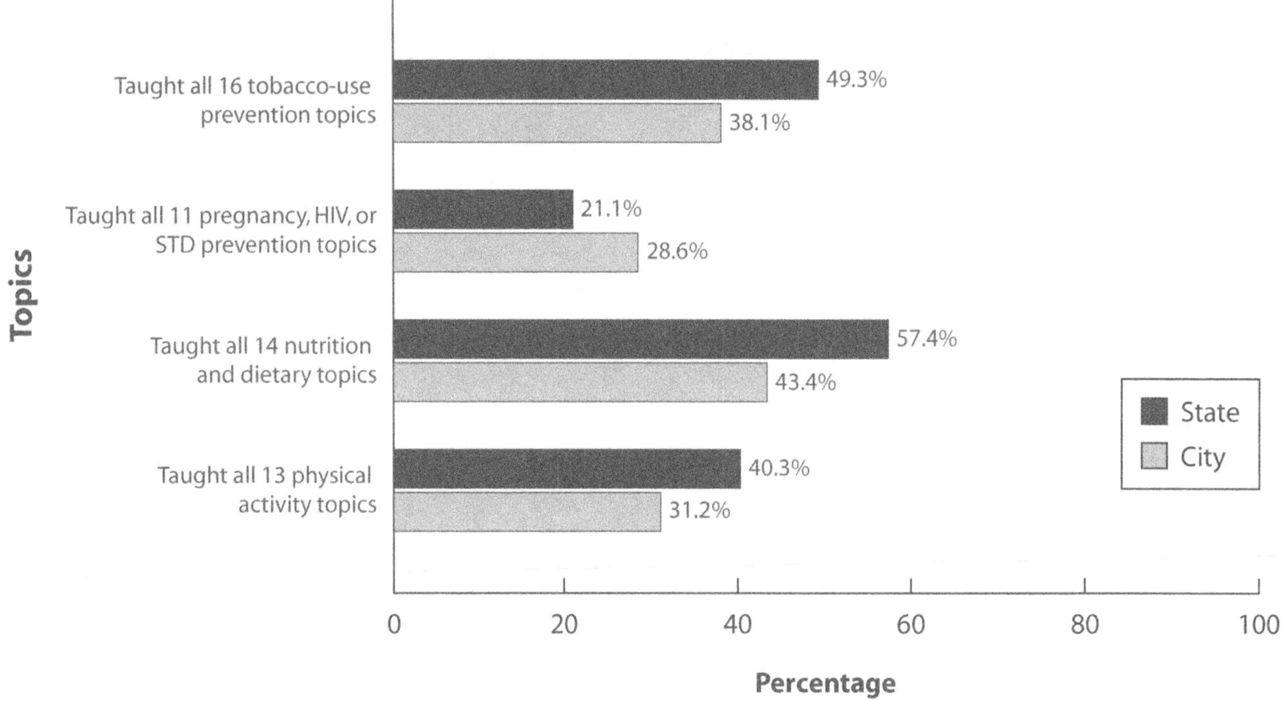

* Human immunodeficiency virus.
† Sexually transmitted disease.

The percentage of all schools that taught all 16 tobacco-use prevention topics in a required health education course during the 2005–2006 school year ranged from 23.1% to 74.5% across states (median: 49.3%) and from 0.0% to 76.8% across cities (median: 38.1%) (Table 12, Figure 2).

Pregnancy, HIV, or STD Prevention Topics

Pregnancy, HIV, or STD prevention topics taught in a required health education course included HIV transmission and prevention; external influences on HIV-related risk behaviors and sexual behaviors; and skills to avoid HIV infection, STDs, and pregnancy. The percentage of all schools that taught about HIV transmission and prevention topics in a required health education course during the 2005–2006 school year ranged as follows (Table 8a):

- **Abstinence as the most effective method to avoid pregnancy, HIV, and STDs:** from 28.5% to 99.3% across states (median: 78.0%) and from 0.0% to 100.0% across cities (median: 56.8%).

- **How HIV is transmitted:** from 28.0% to 99.3% across states (median: 78.7%) and from 0.0% to 100.0% across cities (median: 55.7%).

- **How HIV affects the human body:** from 28.3% to 99.3% across states (median: 77.8%) and from 0.0% to 98.7% across cities (median: 55.7%).

- **Condom efficacy, that is, how well condoms work or do not work:** from 11.7% to 90.0% across states (median: 56.0%) and from 0.0% to 91.1% across cities (median: 53.0%).

- **Risks associated with having multiple sexual partners:** from 26.5% to 96.2% across states (median: 73.7%) and from 0.0% to 95.0% across cities (median: 55.7%).

The percentage of all schools that taught about external influences on HIV-related risk behaviors and sexual behavior; and taught skills to avoid HIV infection, STDs, and pregnancy in a required health education course during the 2005–2006 school year ranged as follows (Table 8b):

- **Influence of alcohol and other drugs on HIV-related risk behaviors:** from 26.8% to 99.3% across states (median: 77.0%) and from 0.0% to 97.4% across cities (median: 54.7%).

- **Social or cultural influences on sexual behavior:** from 63.2% to 87.9% across states (median: 81.8%) and from 0.0% to 90.1% across cities (median: 49.4%).

- **How to prevent HIV infection:** from 27.6% to 98.9% across states (median: 78.2%) and 0.0% to 98.7% across cities (median: 55.7%).

- **How to find valid information or services related to HIV or HIV testing:** from 22.9% to 91.9% across states (median: 64.1%) and from 0.0% to 92.3% across cities (median: 52.9%).

- **How to correctly use a condom:** from 1.0% to 59.1% across states (median: 24.3%) and from 0.0% to 74.8% across cities (median: 34.2%).

- **Compassion for persons living with HIV or AIDS:** from 23.3% to 91.6% across states (median: 65.5%) and from 0.0% to 88.8% across cities (median: 52.4%).

The percentage of all schools that taught all 11 pregnancy, HIV, or STD prevention topics in a required health education course during the 2005–2006 school year ranged from 1.0% to 53.1% across states (median: 21.1%) and from 0.0% to 66.5% across cities (median: 28.6%) (Table 12, Figure 2).

Required HIV Prevention Units or Lessons

Required HIV prevention units or lessons may be taught not only in a required health education course, but also in a variety of other courses. The percentage of all schools that taught required HIV prevention units or lessons in specific courses ranged as follows (Table 9):

- **Science:** from 12.9% to 66.3% across states (median: 32.4%) and from 25.4% to 76.4% across cities (median 53.9%).

- **Home economics or family and consumer education:** from 6.4% to 66.9% across states (median: 24.3%) and from 0.0% to 46.2% across cities (median: 12.0%).

- **Physical education:** from 9.3% to 71.8% across states (median: 26.9%) and from 6.4% to 83.4% across cities (median: 36.7%).

- **Family life education or life skills:** from 14.6% to 86.3% across states (median: 38.3%) and from 28.7% to 71.2% across cities (median: 39.1%).

- **Special education:** from 5.4% to 47.3% across states (median: 16.7%) and from 13.9% to 56.3% across cities (median: 29.4%).

- **Social studies:** from 2.0% to 19.9% across states (median: 7.8%) and from 0.0% to 31.5% across cities (median: 10.0%).

Nutrition and Dietary Behavior Topics

Nutrition and dietary behavior topics taught in a required health education course included choosing healthful foods, food safety, and behaviors that contribute to maintaining a healthy weight. The percentage of all schools that taught about choosing healthful foods in a required health education course during the 2005–2006 school year ranged as follows (Table 10a):

- **Benefits of healthy eating:** from 42.4% to 98.2% across states (median: 84.7%) and from 0.0% to 100.0% across cities (median: 56.8%).
- **Using food labels:** from 37.9% to 95.6% across states (median: 79.4%) and from 0.0% to 98.7% across cities (median: 55.0%).
- **Food guidance using My Pyramid:** from 35.7% to 92.5% across states (median: 77.8%) and from 0.0% to 98.7% across cities (median: 55.0%).
- **Eating more fruits, vegetables, and grain products:** from 41.7% to 97.0% across states (median: 83.3%) and from 0.0% to 100.0% across cities (median: 53.9%).
- **Choosing foods that are low in fat, saturated fat, and cholesterol:** from 40.1% to 96.7% across states (median: 81.3%) and from 0.0% to 98.7% across cities (median: 55.0%).
- **Using sugars in moderation:** from 39.3% to 95.0% across states (median: 80.3%) and from 0.0% to 98.7% across cities (median: 52.9%).
- **Using salt and sodium in moderation:** from 36.0% to 92.9% across states (median: 79.3%) and from 0.0% to 95.1% across cities (median: 53.9%).
- **Eating more calcium-rich foods:** from 37.4% to 92.4% across states (median: 76.3%) and from 0.0% to 94.0% across cities (median: 51.8%).

The percentage of all schools that taught about food safety and behaviors that contribute to maintaining a healthy weight in a required health education course during the 2005–2006 school year ranged as follows (Table 10b):

- **Food safety:** from 33.3% to 93.1% across states (median: 69.6%) and from 0.0% to 89.2% across cities (median: 49.8%).
- **Balancing food intake and physical activity:** from 41.2% to 97.3% across states (median: 83.1%) and from 0.0% to 100.0% across cities (median: 52.1%).
- **Preparing healthy meals and snacks:** from 36.0% to 93.5% across states (median: 74.2%) and from 0.0% to 94.7% across cities (median: 51.2%).
- **Risks of unhealthy weight control practices:** from 38.6% to 97.3% across states (median: 81.6%) and from 0.0% to 98.7% across cities (median: 53.9%).
- **Accepting body size differences:** from 37.1% to 94.4% across states (median: 78.4%) and from 0.0% to 93.9% across cities (median: 55.7%).
- **Eating disorders:** from 36.1% to 95.4% across states (median: 78.5%) and from 0.0% to 95.0% across cities (median: 55.9%).

The percentage of all schools that taught all 14 nutrition and dietary behavior topics in a required health education course during the 2005–2006 school year ranged from 23.8% to 78.0% across states (median: 57.4%) and from 0.0% to 79.2% across cities (median: 43.4%) (Table 12, Figure 2).

Physical Activity Topics

Physical activity topics taught in a required health education course included the benefits of physical activity, guidance for engaging in physical activity, and the challenges to engaging in physical activity. The percentage of all schools that taught about the benefits of physical activity and guidance for engaging in physical activity in a required health education course during the 2005–2006 school year ranged as follows (Table 11a):

- **Physical, psychological, or social benefits of physical activity:** from 41.4% to 96.7% across states (median: 82.6%) and from 0.0% to 92.6% across cities (median: 52.4%).

- **Health-related fitness (i.e., cardiovascular endurance, muscular endurance, muscular strength, flexibility, and body composition):** from 41.3% to 94.5% across states (median: 78.2%) and from 0.0% to 90.1% across cities (median: 50.5%).

- **Difference between physical activity, exercise, and fitness:** from 36.8% to 90.8% across states (median: 73.3%) and from 0.0% to 81.1% across cities (median: 47.9%).

- **Phases of a workout (i.e., warm-up, workout, and cool down):** from 36.8% to 93.2% across states (median: 72.4%) and from 0.0% to 84.6% across cities (median: 45.8%).

- **How much physical activity is enough (i.e., determining frequency, intensity, time, and type of physical activity):** from 35.1% to 92.2% across states (median: 73.3%) and from 0.0% to 86.8% across cities (median: 45.7%).

- **Decreasing sedentary activities such as television watching:** from 40.2% to 93.6% across states (median: 77.2%) and from 0.0% to 92.8% across cities (median: 50.2%).

The percentage of all schools that taught about the challenges to engaging in physical activity in a required health education course during the 2005–2006 school ranged as follows (Table 11b):

- **Overcoming barriers to physical activity:** from 32.6% to 84.2% across states (median: 67.4%) and from 0.0% to 80.6% across cities (median: 46.8%).

- **Developing an individualized physical activity plan:** from 29.1% to 79.6% across states (median: 60.4%) and from 0.0% to 79.3% across cities (median: 41.4%).

- **Monitoring progress toward reaching goals in an individualized physical activity plan:** from 28.9% to 74.8% across states (median: 57.4%) and from 0.0% to 79.5% across cities (median: 38.3%).

- **Opportunities for physical activity in the community:** from 33.0% to 85.9% across states (median: 68.9%) and from 0.0% to 80.0% across cities (median: 43.6%).

- **Preventing injury during physical activity:** from 36.3% to 92.9% across states (median: 72.9%) and from 0.0% to 84.6% across cities (median: 46.9%).

- **Weather-related safety (e.g., avoiding heat stroke, hypothermia, and sunburn while physically active):** from 37.4% to 89.3% across states (median: 71.6%) and from 0.0% to 79.1% across cities (median: 47.0%).

- **Dangers of using performance-enhancing drugs, such as steroids:** from 34.3% to 96.3% across states (median: 78.9%) and from 0.0% to 94.8% across cities (median: 54.7%).

The percentage of all schools that taught all 13 physical activity topics in a required health education course during the 2005–2006 school year ranged from 20.1% to 62.0% across states (median: 40.3%) and from 0.0% to 64.8% across cities (median: 31.2%) (Table 12, Figure 2).

Teaching Methods in Required Health Education Courses

Teachers used a variety of methods to facilitate the learning process. The percentage of all schools that sometimes, almost always, or always used specific teaching methods in a required health education course during the 2005–2006 school year ranged as follows (Table 13a, b):

- **Audio-visual media, such as videos:** from 39.1% to 92.8% across states (median: 79.1%) and from 0.0% to 94.9% across cities (median: 53.2%).

- **Group discussions:** from 42.6% to 97.8% across states (median: 84.7%) and from 0.0% to 100.0% across cities (median: 55.0%).

- **Cooperative group activities:** from 39.9% to 94.3% across states (median: 80.2%) and from 0.0% to 97.7% across cities (median: 52.9%).

- **Role play, simulations, or practice:** from 32.0% to 78.5% across states (median: 58.8%) and from 0.0% to 83.8% across cities (median: 42.9%).

- **Language, performing, or visual arts:** from 23.0% to 66.1% across states (median: 41.0%) and from 0.0% to 76.1% across cities (median: 43.9%).

- **Pledges or contracts for changing behavior or abstaining from a behavior:** from 17.5% to 43.3% across states (median: 28.5%) and from 0.0% to 54.8% across cities (median: 28.0%).

- **Peer teaching:** from 28.7% to 82.7% across states (median: 50.0%) and from 0.0% to 75.2% across cities (median: 42.3%).

- **The Internet:** from 31.5% to 85.4% across states (median: 64.3%) and from 0.0% to 82.9% across cities (median: 39.7%).

- **Computer-assisted instruction:** from 22.5% to 62.4% across states (median: 41.7%) and from 0.0% to 59.1% across cities (median: 27.3%).

- **Guest speakers:** from 29.8% to 77.2% across states (median: 53.0%) and from 0.0% to 64.8% across cities (median: 42.8%).

- **Health education programs available through video-conferencing or other distance learning methods:** from 1.7% to 16.7% across states (median: 7.8%) and from 0.0% to 23.5% across cities (median: 10.0%).

Teachers also used a variety of methods to highlight diversity or the values of various cultures. The percentage of all schools that used specific methods to highlight diversity or the values of various cultures in a required health education course during the 2005–2006 school year ranged as follows (Table 14):

- **Using textbooks or curricular materials reflective of various cultures:** from 31.1% to 72.8% across states (median: 53.5%) and from 0.0% to 87.6% across cities (median: 45.8%).

- **Using textbooks or curricular materials designed for students with limited English proficiency:** from 4.7% to 41.3% across states (median: 22.2%) and from 0.0% to 85.4% across cities (median: 27.2%).

- **Asking students or families to share their own cultural experiences related to health topics:** from

27.7% to 72.3% across states (median: 54.3%) and from 0.0% to 86.7% across cities (median: 44.9%).

- **Teaching about cultural differences and similarities:** from 36.4% to 85.5% across states (median: 65.6%) and from 0.0% to 91.5% across cities (median: 53.9%).

- **Modifying teaching methods to match students' learning styles, health beliefs, or cultural values:** from 40.6% to 92.1% across states (median: 75.3%) and from 0.0% to 97.5% across cities (median: 56.0%).

Coordination of Health Education

The quality of health education may be enhanced by a health education coordinator who coordinates the selection of the curriculum, serves as a content expert for teachers, secures and manages resources, and advocates for school health activities. The percentage of all schools with a health education coordinator ranged from 80.4% to 99.5% across states (median: 95.8%) and from 74.2% to 100.0% across cities (median: 92.7%) (Table 15). Many different staff may serve as the health education coordinator in a school. Among schools with a health education coordinator, the percentage of schools in which specific staff served as the health education coordinator ranged as follows (Table 15):

- **District administrator or district health education or curriculum coordinator:** from 5.9% to 49.0% across states (median: 25.2%) and from 5.8% to 38.1% across cities (median: 19.6%).

- **School administrator:** from 8.5% to 33.9% across states (median: 20.8%) and from 5.9% to 36.9% across cities (median: 13.5%).

- **Health education teacher:** from 24.8% to 75.1% across states (median: 46.9%) and from 14.6% to 63.7% across cities (median: 49.3%).

- **School nurse:** from 0.0% to 8.7% across states (median: 2.1%) and from 0.0% to 9.1% across cities (median: 2.7%).

- **Someone else:** from 1.1% to 14.2% across states (median: 3.8%) and from 0.0% to 29.8% across cities (median: 10.1%).

During the 2005–2006 school year, health education staff worked on health education activities with other school staff. The percentage of all schools in which health education staff worked on health education activities with others ranged as follows (Table 16):

- **Physical education staff:** from 54.6% to 91.1% across states (median: 76.7%) and from 45.1% to 96.8% across cities (median: 59.9%).

- **School health services staff (e.g., nurses):** from 28.2% to 87.8% across states (median: 66.4%) and from 26.2% to 84.8% across cities (median: 67.6%).

- **School mental health or social services staff (e.g., psychologists, counselors, and social workers):** from 38.3% to 82.4% across states (median: 55.8%) and from 22.9% to 87.5% across cities (median: 56.3%).

- **Nutrition or food service staff:** from 13.5% to 49.4% across states (median: 37.9%) and from 8.5% to 54.3% across cities (median: 27.5%).

Professional Preparation and Staff Development

Lead health education teachers reported professional preparation in many disciplines. The percentage of all schools in which the major emphasis of the lead health education teacher's professional preparation was in each specific discipline ranged as follows (Table 17):

- **Health and physical education combined:** from 9.5% to 88.9% across states (median: 45.5%) and from 1.8% to 85.0% across cities (median: 26.4%).

- **Health education only:** from 1.2% to 42.9% across states (median: 4.7%) and from 0.0% to 37.1% across cities (median: 8.0%).

- **Physical education only:** from 2.0% to 36.4% across states (median: 11.8%) and from 0.0% to 24.5% across cities (median: 8.6%).

- **Other education degree:** from 0.0% to 33.7% across states (median: 5.2%) and from 0.0% to 26.7% across cities (median: 4.6%).

- **Kinesiology, exercise science or exercise physiology, home economics or family and consumer science, biology, or other science:** from 0.0% to 28.6% across states (median: 10.7%) and from 0.0% to 55.1% across cities (median: 11.0%).

- **Nursing or counseling:** from 0.0% to 18.2% across states (median: 2.7%) and from 0.0% to 85.4% across cities (median: 2.7%).

- **Public health, nutrition, or another discipline:** from 0.0% to 14.4% across states (median: 2.9%) and from 0.0% to 18.4% across cities (median: 3.2%).

The percentage of all schools that required newly hired staff who teach health topics to be certified, licensed, or endorsed by the state in health education ranged from 23.8% to 99.0% across states (median: 84.5%) and from 0.0% to 100.0% across cities (median: 75.7%) (Table 18).

The percentage of all schools in which the lead health education teacher was certified, licensed, or endorsed by their state to teach health education in middle school or high school ranged from 26.7% to 97.7% across states (median: 79.6%) and from 35.3% to 91.7% across cities (median: 69.4%) (Table 18).

The percentage of all schools in which the lead health education teacher had experience teaching health education classes or topics for a specific number of years ranged as follows (Table 18):

- **1 year:** from 1.7% to 23.1% across states (median: 7.5%) and from 2.4% to 29.4% across cities (median: 9.9%).

- **2 to 5 years:** from 12.4% to 38.4% across states (median: 22.9%) and from 12.6% to 48.5% across cities (median: 22.7%).

- **6 to 9 years:** from 12.1% to 23.8% across states (median: 16.6%) and from 1.9% to 32.7% across cities (median: 15.5%).

- **10 to 14 years:** from 9.7% to 22.5% across states (median: 13.8%) and from 0.0% to 27.5% across cities (median: 13.9%).

- **15 years or more:** from 16.2% to 59.4% across states (median: 37.9%) and from 8.8% to 63.1% across cities (median: 36.0%).

Lead health education teachers received staff development during the 2 years preceding the survey on many health topics. The percentage of all schools in which the lead health education teacher received staff development on specific topics ranged as follows (Tables 19a, b, c):

- **Alcohol-use or other drug-use prevention:** from 36.3% to 70.0% across states (median: 50.4%) and from 39.0% to 100.0% across cities (median: 64.5%).

- **Asthma awareness:** from 11.0% to 57.4% across states (median: 19.2%) and from 5.9% to 68.0% across cities (median: 33.8%).

- **Consumer health:** from 14.0% to 42.2% across states (median: 22.2%) and from 17.2% to 53.3% across cities (median: 27.7%).
- **CPR:** from 29.6% to 85.4% across states (median: 67.0%) and from 38.2% to 88.0% across cities (median: 58.1%).
- **Dental and oral health:** from 3.5% to 22.7% across states (median: 12.3%) and from 5.0% to 37.3% across cities (median: 14.4%).
- **Emotional and mental health:** from 23.8% to 62.3% across states (median: 35.6%) and from 18.4% to 86.7% across cities (median: 45.3%).
- **Environmental health:** from 7.7% to 21.4% across states (median: 14.2%) and from 7.5% to 38.9% across cities (median: 20.4%).
- **First aid:** from 29.1% to 77.1% across states (median: 56.7%) and from 24.3% to 90.0% across cities (median: 50.7%).
- **Foodborne illness prevention:** from 9.2% to 30.2% across states (median: 18.9%) and from 6.1% to 38.5% across cities (median: 18.8%).
- **Growth and development:** from 17.9% to 49.8% across states (median: 25.7%) and from 21.2% to 65.4% across cities (median: 47.2%).
- **HIV prevention:** from 21.3% to 63.9% across states (median: 43.7%) and from 42.9% to 100.0% across cities (median: 64.2%).
- **Human sexuality:** from 12.7% to 65.6% across states (median: 31.6%) and from 32.2% to 100.0% across cities (median: 63.8%).
- **Immunizations:** from 7.4% to 30.7% across states (median: 16.6%) and from 6.1% to 36.9% across cities (median: 22.7%).
- **Injury prevention and safety:** from 25.0% to 58.6% across states (median: 39.9%) and from 24.5% to 75.8% across cities (median: 41.9%).
- **Nutrition and dietary behavior:** from 21.3% to 72.8% across states (median: 35.4%) and from 21.8% to 63.6% across cities (median: 43.4%).
- **Physical activity and fitness:** from 27.5% to 64.6% across states (median: 48.3%) and from 23.6% to 81.2% across cities (median: 46.9%).
- **Pregnancy prevention:** from 10.3% to 55.7% across states (median: 27.5%) and from 22.9% to 92.8% across cities (median: 42.6%).
- **STD prevention:** from 17.4% to 64.8% across states (median: 36.7%) and from 35.4% to 100.0% across cities (median: 58.7%).
- **Suicide prevention:** from 11.4% to 39.6% across states (median: 25.5%) and from 16.3% to 82.8% across cities (median: 31.0%).
- **Sun safety or skin cancer prevention:** from 6.8% to 43.1% across states (median: 13.4%) and from 6.1% to 46.1% across cities (median: 18.4%).
- **Tobacco-use prevention:** from 16.7% to 49.7% across states (median: 34.6%) and from 28.1% to 100.0% across cities (median: 40.7%).
- **Violence prevention:** from 40.7% to 70.1% across states (median: 52.3%) and from 44.0% to 81.4% across cities (median: 64.8%).

The percentage of all schools in which the lead health education teacher wanted to receive staff development on specific health topics ranged as follows (Tables 20a, b, c):

- **Alcohol-use or other drug-use prevention:** from 53.7% to 81.4% across states (median: 72.5%) and from 48.3% to 85.9% across cities (median: 75.4%).

- **Asthma awareness:** from 33.0% to 68.3% across states (median: 56.5%) and from 35.3% to 85.2% across cities (median: 66.2%).

- **Consumer health:** from 36.1% to 65.5% across states (median: 49.4%) and from 35.2% to 74.5% across cities (median: 60.3%).

- **CPR:** from 48.9% to 78.4% across states (median: 64.4%) and from 60.6% to 84.6% across cities (median: 74.8%).

- **Dental and oral health:** from 27.0% to 57.4% across states (median: 42.5%) and from 33.6% to 76.3% across cities (median: 52.4%).

- **Emotional and mental health:** from 55.6% to 80.2% across states (median: 67.4%) and from 62.9% to 87.5% across cities (median: 77.7%).

- **Environmental health:** from 37.1% to 65.9% across states (median: 52.5%) and from 38.6% to 80.6% across cities (median: 61.1%).

- **First aid:** from 50.2% to 79.6% across states (median: 65.1%) and from 56.8% to 84.4% across cities (median: 73.6%).

- **Foodborne illness prevention:** from 35.8% to 61.4% across states (median: 49.8%) and from 39.4% to 80.6% across cities (median: 61.3%).

- **Growth and development:** from 39.4% to 67.0% across states (median: 55.9%) and from 47.3% to 83.8% across cities (median: 64.8%).

- **HIV prevention:** from 46.1% to 77.4% across states (median: 63.5%) and from 60.5% to 84.6% across cities (median: 70.1%).

- **Human sexuality:** from 40.9% to 75.4% across states (median: 57.3%) and from 50.5% to 80.6% across cities (median: 69.1%).

- **Immunizations:** from 30.7% to 59.5% across states (median: 45.1%) and from 33.8% to 80.3% across cities (median: 55.8%).

- **Injury prevention and safety:** from 42.0% to 72.4% across states (median: 59.6%) and from 42.5% to 78.6% across cities (median: 64.3%).

- **Nutrition and dietary behavior:** from 57.3% to 78.5% across states (median: 73.2%) and from 58.5% to 83.1% across cities (median: 76.3%).

- **Physical activity and fitness:** from 50.9% to 78.5% across states (median: 67.8%) and from 46.8% to 83.8% across cities (median: 67.3%).

- **Pregnancy prevention:** from 39.5% to 72.3% across states (median: 57.9%) and from 49.3% to 84.4% across cities (median: 67.1%).

- **STD prevention:** from 46.2% to 77.7% across states (median: 62.8%) and from 55.1% to 88.0% across cities (median: 70.0%).

- **Suicide prevention:** from 62.6% to 85.2% across states (median: 72.3%) and from 62.9% to 96.3% across cities (median: 77.2%).

- **Sun safety or skin cancer prevention:** from 40.0% to 66.1% across states (median: 55.9%) and from 42.8% to 73.8% across cities (median: 60.0%).

- **Tobacco-use prevention:** from 45.1% to 74.3% across states (median: 63.5%) and from 51.5% to 83.8% across cities (median: 66.0%).

- **Violence prevention:** from 58.7% to 83.6% across states (median: 76.3%) and from 63.4% to 94.8% across cities (median: 82.5%).

Lead health education teachers also received staff development during the two years preceding the survey on specific teaching topics. The percentage of all schools in which the lead health education teacher had received staff development on specific topics ranged as follows (Table 21):

- **Teaching students with physical, medical, or cognitive disabilities:** from 35.1% to 64.9% across states (median: 49.6%) and from 24.9% to 73.6% across cities (median: 41.1%).

- **Teaching students of various cultural backgrounds:** from 12.5% to 65.9% across states (median: 39.6%) and from 21.7% to 77.5% across cities (median: 60.1%).

- **Teaching students with limited English proficiency:** from 7.6% to 77.9% across states (median: 25.9%) and from 17.5% to 85.6% across cities (median: 49.5%).

- **Using interactive teaching methods such as role plays or cooperative group activities:** from 35.7% to 68.0% across states (median: 52.1%) and from 52.3% to 89.8% across cities (median: 65.0%).

- **Encouraging family or community involvement:** from 26.1% to 72.0% across states (median: 36.9%) and from 32.6% to 73.1% across cities (median: 53.0%).

- **Teaching skills for behavior change:** from 31.6% to 61.1% across states (median: 46.2%) and from 35.8% to 78.0% across cities (median: 61.0%).

- **Classroom management techniques, such as social skills training, environmental modification, conflict resolution and mediation, and behavior management:** from 39.4% to 75.7% across states (median: 57.1%) and from 49.7% to 90.2% across cities (median: 61.8%).

- **Assessing or evaluating students in health education:** from 15.2% to 66.7% across states (median: 31.4%) and from 25.8% to 82.2% across cities (median: 32.4%).

The percentage of all schools in which the lead health education teacher wanted to receive staff development on specific teaching methods ranged as follows (Table 22):

- **Teaching students with physical, medical, or cognitive disabilities:** from 49.8% to 72.9% across states (median: 63.8%) and from 45.2% to 90.2% across cities (median: 72.4%).

- **Teaching students of various cultural backgrounds:** from 36.5% to 66.8% across states (median: 58.2%) and from 43.6% to 85.8% across cities (median: 69.2%).

- **Teaching students with limited English proficiency:** from 30.7% to 65.0% across states (median: 53.8%) and from 42.7% to 81.4% across cities (median: 64.6%).

FIGURE 3. Median percentage of schools that taught a required physical education course in each grade,* School Health Profiles, 2006.

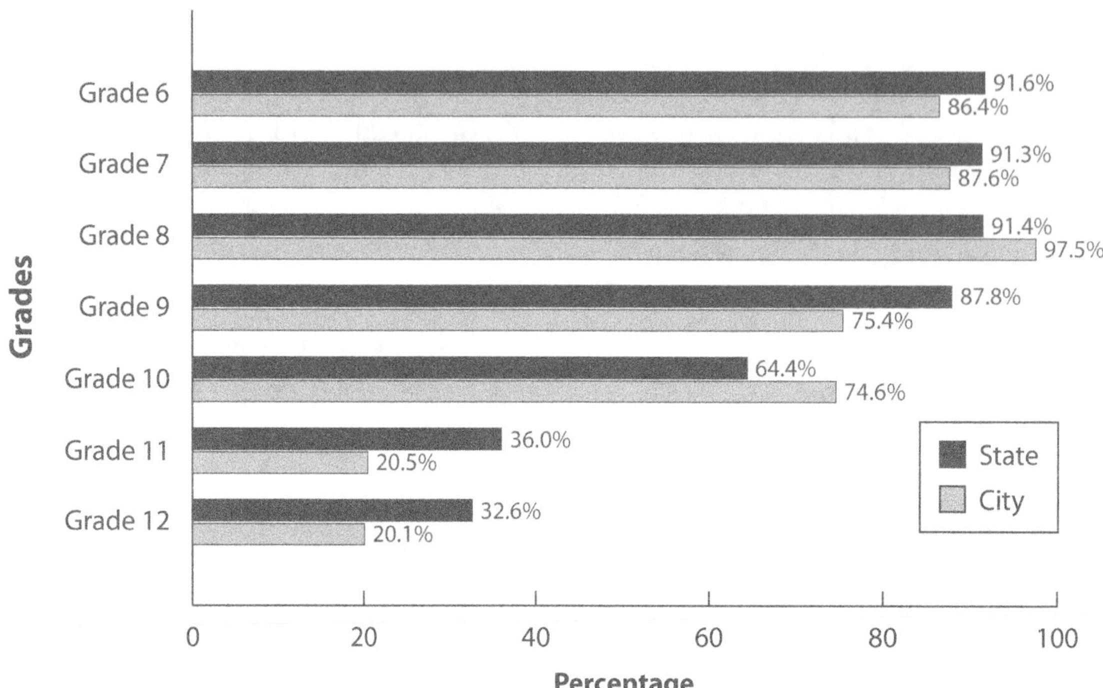

* Among schools with students in each grade.

- **Using interactive teaching methods such as role plays or cooperative group activities:** from 44.7% to 72.1% across states (median: 61.3%) and from 46.5% to 81.9% across cities (median: 68.1%).

- **Encouraging family or community involvement:** from 53.6% to 72.4% across states (median: 64.0%) and from 50.7% to 87.7% across cities (median: 72.7%).

- **Teaching skills for behavior change:** from 65.2% to 85.7% across states (median: 72.8%) and from 63.2% to 91.0% across cities (median: 78.8%).

- **Classroom management techniques:** from 52.4% to 75.7% across states (median: 67.1%) and from 58.0% to 89.3% across cities (median: 75.6%).

- **Assessing or evaluating students in health education:** from 58.6% to 83.2% across states (median: 68.8%) and from 48.9% to 91.8% across cities (median: 72.7%).

PHYSICAL EDUCATION AND PHYSICAL ACTIVITY

Required Physical Education

Physical education is defined on the Profiles questionnaire as instruction that helps students develop the knowledge, attitudes, motor skills, behavioral skills, and confidence needed to adopt and maintain a physically active lifestyle. Many schools required physical education for students in grades 6 through 12. The percentage of all schools that required physical education for students in any of grades 6 through 12 ranged from 36.8% to 100.0% across states (median: 97.3%) and from 44.0% to 100.0% across cities (median: 95.6%) (Table 23).

A required physical education course is taught as a semester-long, quarter-long, or year-long unit of instruction for which the student receives credit. It is *not* recess, intramural activities, physical activity clubs, or school sports. The percentage of all schools that required students to take only one required physical education course ranged from 4.8% to 47.4% across states (median: 18.1%) and from 4.7% to 47.3% across cities (median: 27.5%) (Table 23). The percentage of all schools that required students to take two or more required physical education courses ranged from 14.4% to 94.6% across states (median: 76.6%) and from 30.9% to 93.9% across cities (median: 61.1%) (Table 23).

Among schools that required a physical education course for students in any of grades 6 through 12, some schools required that students who fail the course repeat it. The percentage of these schools that required students to repeat a required physical education course ranged from 37.9% to 80.6% across states (median: 55.6%) and from 26.4% to 82.7% across cities (median: 52.1%) (Table 23).

The percentage of all schools that required newly hired staff who teach physical education to be certified, licensed, or endorsed by the state in physical education ranged from 35.0% to 100.0% across states (median: 97.0%) and from 90.6% to 100.0% across cities (median: 98.3%) (Table 23).

Among schools with students in particular grades, the percentage of schools across states that taught a required physical education course in that grade ranged from 9.9% to 100.0% (median: 91.6%) in grade 6, 7.8% to 100.0% (median: 91.3%) in grade 7, 9.2% to 100.0% (median: 91.4%) in grade 8, 23.3% to 100.0% (median: 87.8%) in grade 9, 12.8% to 98.9% (median: 64.4%) in grade 10, 5.4% to 100.0% (median: 36.0%) in grade 11, and from 5.4% to 98.9% (median: 32.6%) in grade 12 (Table 24, Figure 3). Among schools with students in particular grades, the percentage of schools across cities that taught a required physical education course in that grade ranged from 14.3% to 100.0% (median: 86.4%) in grade 6, 14.3% to 100.0% (median: 87.6%) in grade 7, 14.3% to 100.0% (median: 87.5%) in grade 8, 38.3% to 100.0% (median: 75.4%) in grade 9, 21.2% to 93.7% (median: 74.6%) in grade 10, 17.3% to 77.4% (median: 20.5%) in grade 11, and from 16.0% to 77.4% (median: 20.1%) in grade 12 (Table 24, Figure 3).

Among schools that required a physical education course for students in any of grades 6 through 12, the percentage of schools that allowed students to be exempted from taking a required physical education course for specific reasons ranged as follows (Table 25a, b):

- **Religious reasons:** from 16.3% to 64.5% across states (median: 37.1%) and from 27.5% to 67.9% across cities (median: 43.9%).
- **Long-term physical or medical disability:** from 63.1% to 92.7% across states (median: 79.7%) and from 47.9% to 92.6% across cities (median: 77.4%).
- **Cognitive disability:** from 11.5% to 59.8% across states (median: 28.1%) and from 12.7% to 47.2% across cities (median: 32.5%).
- **Enrollment in other courses (i.e., math or science):** from 0.0% to 48.7% across states (median: 15.2%) and from 5.1% to 49.0% across cities (median: 14.6%).
- **Participation in school sports:** from 0.5% to 75.4% across states (median: 5.4%) and from 0.0% to 73.2% across cities (median: 23.2%).
- **Participation in other school activities (i.e., ROTC, band, or chorus):** from 0.0% to 56.9% across states (median: 8.9%) and from 7.7% to 64.8% across cities (median: 39.6%).

FIGURE 4. Median percentage of all schools that allowed use of physical activity or athletic facilities* or that offered opportunities for students to participate in intramural activities or physical activity clubs, School Health Profiles 2006.

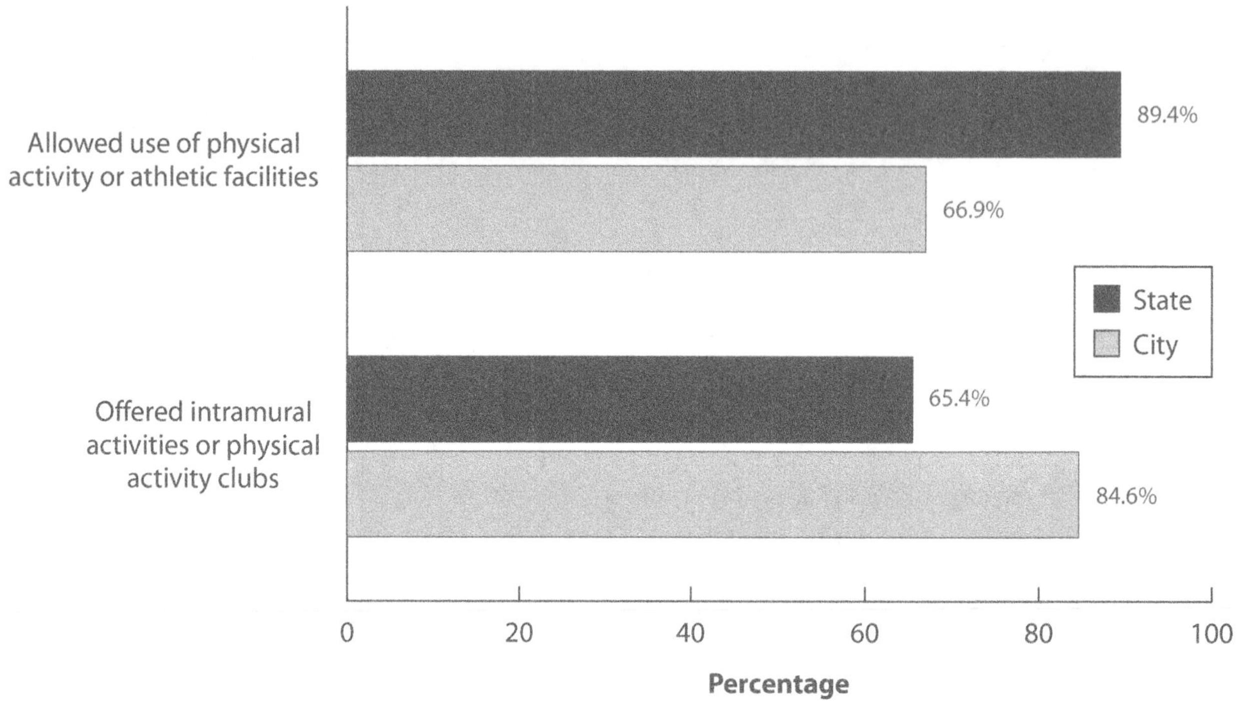

* For community-sponsored sports teams, classes, or lessons outside of school hours or when school is not in session.

- **Participation in community sports activities:** from 0.0% to 16.8% across states (median: 2.0%) and from 0.0% to 15.3% across cities (median: 3.3%).

- **High physical fitness competency test score:** from 0.0% to 17.4% across states (median: 0.8%) and from 0.0% to 14.7% across cities (median: 1.6%).

- **Participation in vocational training:** from 0.0% to 25.7% across states (median: 2.5%) and from 0.0% to 23.8% across cities (median: 1.8%).

- **Participation in community service activities:** from 0.0% to 11.0% across states (median: 1.2%) and from 0.0% to 3.8% across cities (median: 1.5%).

The percentage of schools that did not allow students in any of grades 6 through 12 to be exempted from a required physical education course for enrollment in other courses, participation in school sports, participation in other school activities, participation in community sports activities, high physical fitness competency test scores, participation in vocational training, and participation in community service activities ranged from 17.0% to 95.2% across states (median: 71.3%) and from 12.7% to 83.6% across cities (median: 44.1%).

Physical Activity

Schools can promote physical activity among students by supporting walking or biking to and from school and by allowing community-sponsored sports teams or physical activity programs to use school facilities outside of school hours or when school is not in session. The percentage of all schools that supported or promoted walking or biking to and from school (e.g., through promotional activities, designating safe routes or preferred routes, or having storage facilities for bicycles and helmets) ranged from 10.3% to 62.9% across states (median: 46.1%) and from 18.1% to 80.8% across cities (median: 42.1%). The percentage of all schools that allowed use of their physical activity or athletic facilities for community-sponsored sports teams, classes, or lessons outside of school hours or when school is not in session ranged from 64.0% to 97.6% across states (median: 89.4%) and from 58.0% to 98.9% across cities (median: 66.9%) (Table 26, Figure 4).

Schools also may offer students the opportunity to participate in intramural activities or physical activity clubs. The percentage of all schools that offered opportunities for students to participate in intramural activities or physical activity clubs ranged from 35.4% to 90.1% across states (median: 65.4%) and from 61.9% to 95.0% across cities (median: 84.6%) (Table 26, Figure 4). Among those schools, the percentage that provided transportation home for students who participated in after-school intramural activities or physical activity clubs ranged from 10.3% to 76.5% among states (median: 30.8%) and from 6.8% to 68.0% across cities (median: 19.9%) (Table 26).

NUTRITION SERVICES

Most schools serve lunch to their students. The percentage of all schools that served lunch ranged from 88.9% to 100.0% across states (median: 99.6%) and from 96.0% to 100.0% across cities (median: 100.0%) (Table 27). It is important that students have enough time to eat lunch once they are seated. Among schools that served lunch to students, the percentage of schools in which students usually had 20 minutes or more to eat lunch once they were seated ranged from 64.7% to 95.9% across states (median: 82.8%) and from 58.5% to 94.4% across cities (median: 78.5%) (Table 27).

HEALTHY AND SAFE SCHOOL ENVIRONMENT

Competitive Foods

The percentage of all schools that allowed students to purchase snack foods or beverages from one or more vending machines at the school or at a school store, canteen, or snack bar ranged from 61.9% to 94.0% across states (median: 83.3%) and from 31.5% to 88.6% across cities (median: 79.2%) (Table 28a, b; Figure 5).

The percentage of all schools that allowed students to purchase less nutritious snack foods and beverages from vending machines or at the school store, canteen, or snack bar ranged as follows (Table 28a, Figure 5):

- **2% or whole milk (plain or flavored):** from 15.9% to 67.9% across states (median: 43.4%) and from 16.1% to 64.6% across cities (median: 41.5%).

- **Chocolate candy:** from 8.4% to 82.9% across states (median: 40.3%) and from 4.0% to 59.1% across cities (median: 24.1%).

- **Other kinds of candy:** from 11.2% to 82.6% across states (median: 43.6%) and from 5.7% to 59.3% across cities (median: 28.3%).

- **Salty snacks that are not low in fat, such as regular potato chips:** from 11.0% to 75.9% across states (median: 47.4%) and from 4.4% to 81.0% across cities (median: 42.2%).

- **Soda pop or fruit drinks that are not 100% juice:** from 25.3% to 86.0% across states (median: 62.5%) and from 9.6% to 71.9% across cities (median: 52.4%).

- **Sports drinks:** from 30.5% to 90.2% across states (median: 72.7%) and from 18.0% to 84.3% across cities (median: 71.6%).

FIGURE 5. Median percentage of all schools that allowed students to purchase less nutritious and more nutritious snack foods or beverages, School Health Profiles, 2006.

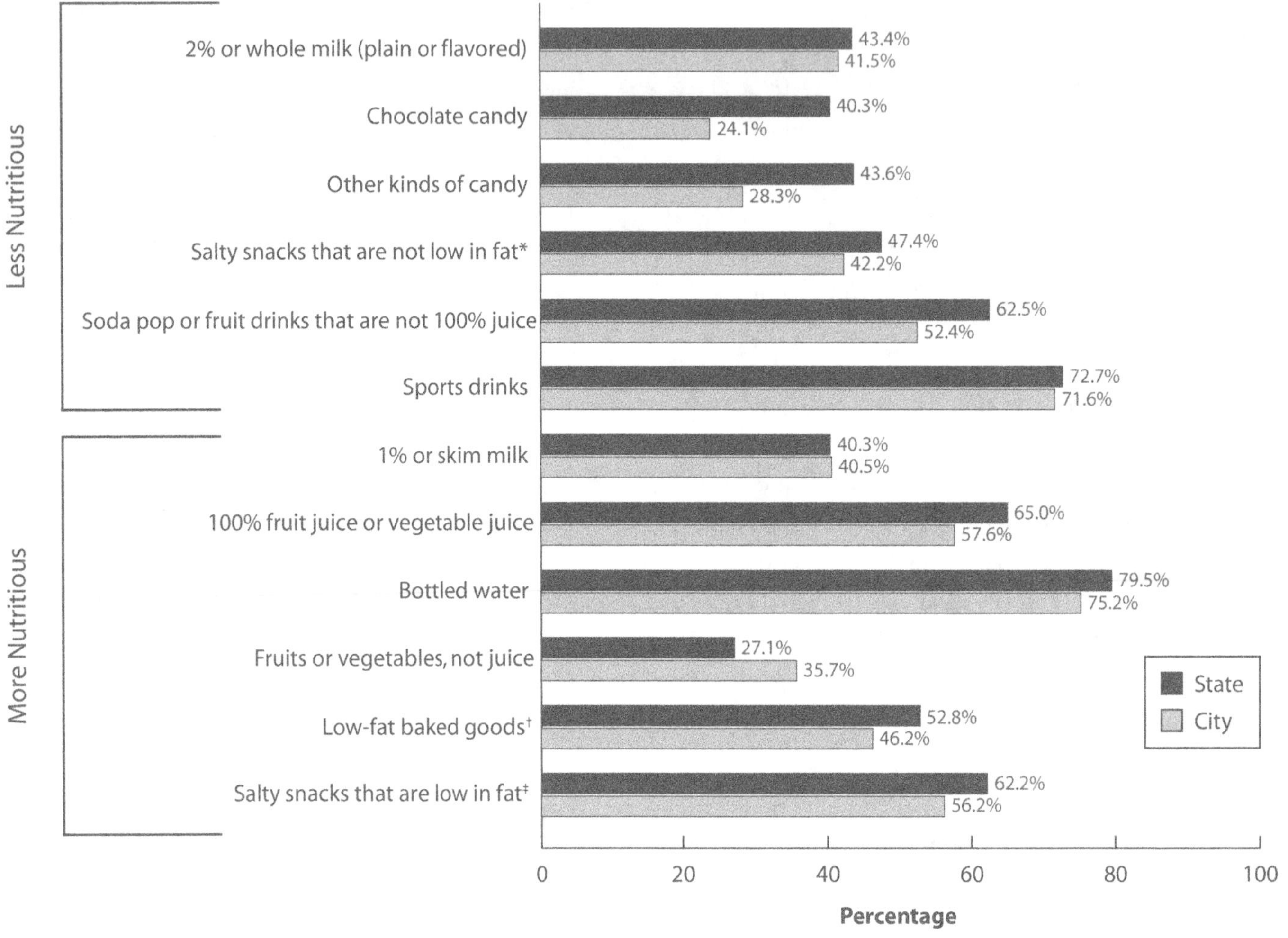

* Such as regular potato chips.

† Such as cookies, crackers, cakes, pastries, or other low-fat baked goods.

‡ Such as pretzels, baked chips, or other low fat chips.

The percentage of all schools that allowed students to purchase more nutritious snack foods and beverages from vending machines or at the school store, canteen, or snack bar ranged as follows (Table 28b, Figure 5):

- **1% or skim milk:** from 10.7% to 66.2% across states (median: 40.3%) and from 14.7% to 60.1% across cities (median: 40.5%).
- **100% fruit juice or vegetable juice:** from 41.0% to 78.6% across states (median: 65.0%) and from 25.0% to 75.9% across cities (median: 57.6%).
- **Bottled water:** from 55.6% to 90.8% across states (median: 79.5%) and from 29.0% to 86.6% across cities (median: 75.2%).
- **Fruits or vegetables, not juice:** from 6.6% to 46.8% across states (median: 27.1%) and from 10.3% to 58.8% across cities (median: 35.7%).

- **Low-fat cookies, crackers, cakes, pastries, or other low-fat baked goods:** from 9.8% to 73.4% across states (median: 52.8%) and from 13.4% to 69.2% across cities (median: 46.2%).

- **Salty snacks that are low in fat, such as pretzels, baked chips, or other low-fat chips:** from 12.5% to 82.9% across states (median: 62.2%) and from 14.2% to 81.0% across cities (median: 56.2%).

The percentage of all schools that allowed students to purchase candy; snacks that are not low in fat; soda pop, sports drinks, or fruit drinks that are not 100% fruit juice; or 2% or whole milk during specific times of the school day ranged as follows (Table 29):

- **Before classes begin in the morning:** from 20.2% to 72.5% across states (median: 35.0%) and from 7.2% to 58.0% across cities (median: 27.6%).

- **During any school hours when meals are not being served:** from 11.9% to 56.6% across states (median: 29.3%) and from 2.9% to 39.1% across cities (median: 12.0%).

- **During school lunch periods:** from 3.9% to 81.3% across states (median: 34.9%) and from 15.7% to 72.3% across cities (median: 36.9%).

The percentage of all schools that had a policy stating that if food is served at student parties, after-school or extended day programs, or concession stands, fruits or vegetables would be among the foods offered ranged from 9.9% to 38.0% across states (median: 17.9%) and from 8.7% to 62.3% across cities (median: 23.1%) (Table 29).

Tobacco-Use Prevention

Policies prohibiting tobacco use at school can help prevent tobacco use among students. The percentage of all schools that had a policy prohibiting tobacco use ranged from 94.3% to 100.0% across states (median: 98.9%) and from 84.0% to 100.0% across cities (median: 98.2%) (Table 30). The percentage of all schools that prohibited the use of all tobacco, including cigarettes, smokeless tobacco (i.e., chewing tobacco, snuff, or dip), cigars, and pipes; by students, faculty and school staff, and visitors; in school buildings, outside on school grounds (including parking lots and playing fields), on school buses or other vehicles used to transport students, and at off-campus, school-sponsored events; ranged from 22.8% to 76.3% across states (median: 53.8%) and from 15.5% to 79.5% across cities (median: 56.0%) (Table 30, Figure 6).

Among schools with a policy prohibiting tobacco use, specific actions may be taken when students are caught smoking cigarettes. The percentage of these schools that sometimes, almost always, or always took specific actions when students were caught smoking cigarettes ranged as follows (Tables 31a, b):

- **Informed parents or guardians:** from 93.2% to 100.0% across states (median: 98.3%) and from 82.5% to 100.0% across cities (median: 97.0%).

- **Referred students to a school counselor:** from 57.1% to 92.1% across states (median: 76.9%) and from 65.6% to 98.2% across cities (median: 84.9%).

- **Referred students to a school administrator:** from 92.6% to 100.0% across states (median: 97.9%) and from 81.1% to 100.0% across cities (median: 94.6%).

- **Encouraged, but not required, students to participate in an assistance, education, or cessation program:** from 30.3% to 81.2% across states (median: 60.2%) and from 38.7% to 90.7% across cities (median: 65.7%).

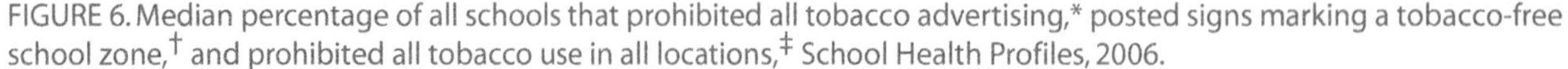

FIGURE 6. Median percentage of all schools that prohibited all tobacco advertising,* posted signs marking a tobacco-free school zone,† and prohibited all tobacco use in all locations,‡ School Health Profiles, 2006.

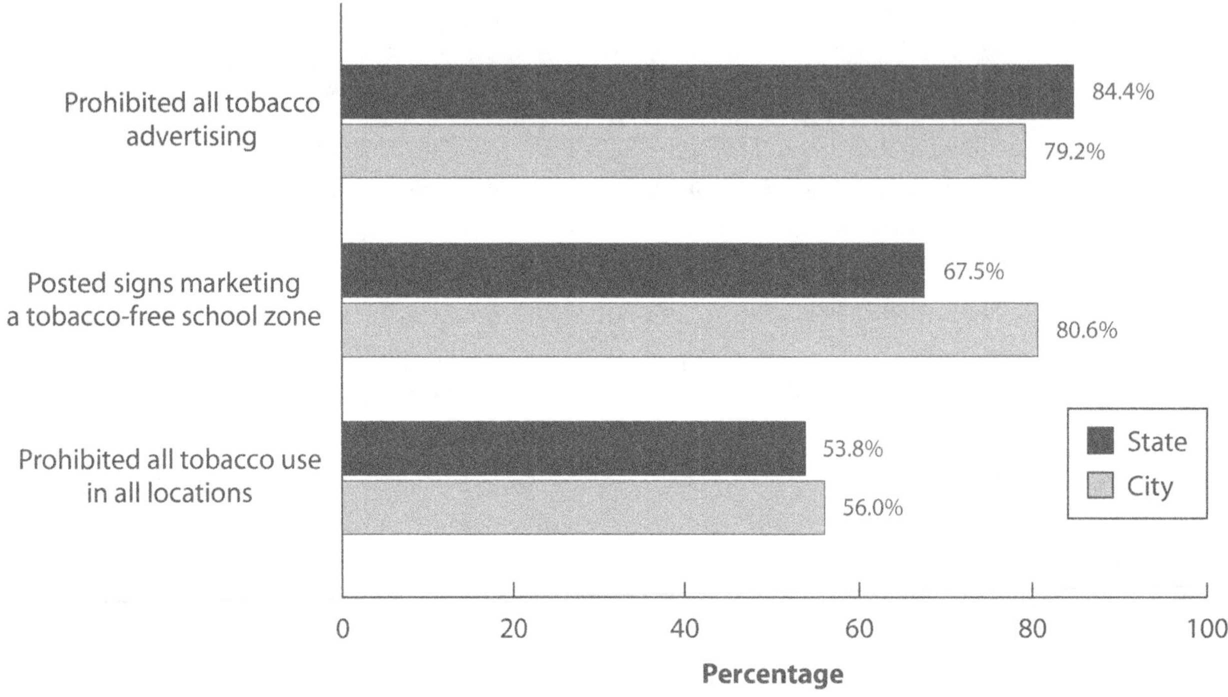

* In school buildings, on school grounds, on school buses and other school vehicles, in school publications, and through sponsorship of school events; and prohibited students from wearing tobacco brand-name apparel or carrying merchandise with tobacco company names, logos, or cartoon characters.

† A specified distance from school grounds where tobacco use is not allowed.

‡ Prohibited the use of all tobacco, including cigarettes, smokeless tobacco (i.e., chewing tobacco, snuff, or dip), cigars, and pipes; by students, faculty and school staff, and visitors; in school buildings, outside on school grounds (including parking lots and playing fields), on school buses or other vehicles used to transport students, and at off-campus school-sponsored events.

- **Required students to participate in an assistance, education, or cessation program:** from 10.3% to 70.4% across states (median: 32.7%) and from 18.2% to 84.7% across cities (median: 48.6%).
- **Referred students to legal authorities:** from 15.4% to 97.2% across states (median: 58.0%) and from 19.3% to 75.4% across cities (median: 48.5%).
- **Placed students in detention:** from 50.9% to 84.4% across states (median: 62.7%) and from 52.2% to 87.0% across cities (median: 66.7%).
- **Gave students in-school suspension:** from 54.7% to 89.7% across states (median: 69.0%) and from 54.7% to 93.3% across cities (median: 69.7%).
- **Did not allow students to participate in extracurricular activities or interscholastic sports:** from 49.9% to 97.7% across states (median: 74.4%) and from 36.9% to 64.0% across cities (median: 55.3%).
- **Suspended students from school:** from 53.2% to 89.0% across states (median: 75.4%) and from 56.4% to 92.8% across cities (median: 75.1%).

- **Expelled students from school:** from 0.0% to 18.9% across states (median: 8.3%) and from 0.0% to 24.2% across cities (median: 9.7%).

- **Reassigned students to an alternative school:** from 0.6% to 37.7% across states (median: 7.3%) and from 0.0% to 31.6% across cities (median: 14.2%).

Among schools with a policy prohibiting tobacco use, the percentage of these schools that had procedures to inform specific groups about the tobacco-use prevention policy that prohibited their use of tobacco ranged from 97.6% to 100.0% across states (median: 99.5%) and from 95.8% to 100.0% across cities (median: 98.0%) for students, from 90.6% to 99.4% across states (median: 96.4%) and from 81.3% to 100.0% across cities (median: 96.4%) for faculty and staff, and from 74.0% to 96.6% across states (median: 87.3%) and from 69.5% to 96.0% across cities (median 86.7%) for visitors (Table 32).

In addition, among schools with a policy prohibiting tobacco use, the percentage of these schools that had a policy to inform students' families about the rules related to tobacco use by students ranged from 95.2% to 100.0% across states (median: 98.7%) and from 90.9% to 100.0% across cities (median: 95.3%) (Table 32).

Many schools prohibit tobacco advertisements in specific locations, tobacco advertising through sponsorship of school events, and students from wearing tobacco brand-name apparel or carrying merchandise with tobacco company names, logos, or cartoon characters. The percentage of all schools that implemented such policies ranged as follows (Table 33):

- **Prohibited tobacco advertising in the school building:** from 92.1% o 100.0% across states (median: 95.4%) and from 90.3% to 100.0% across cities (median: 93.7%).

- **Prohibited tobacco advertising on school grounds, including on the outside of the school building, on playing fields, or other areas of the campus:** from 90.8% to 100.0% across states (median: 94.7%) and from 87.2% to 100.0% across cities (median: 92.4%).

- **Prohibited tobacco advertising on school buses or other vehicles used to transport students:** from 91.3% to 98.5% across states (median: 94.7%) and from 84.7% to 98.2% across cities (median: 92.3%).

- **Prohibited tobacco advertising in school publications (e.g., newsletters, newspapers, web sites, or other school publications):** from 90.6% to 98.6% across states (median: 93.7%) and from 87.4% to 98.2% across cities (median: 91.6%).

- **Prohibited tobacco advertising through sponsorship of school events:** from 89.3% to 95.9% across states (median: 92.7%) and from 80.8% to 97.5% across cities (median: 90.6%).

- **Prohibited students from wearing tobacco brand-name apparel or carrying merchandise with tobacco company names, logos, or cartoon characters:** from 78.2% to 98.9% across states (median: 95.7%) and from 71.6% to 100.0% across cities (median: 91.5%).

- **Prohibited all tobacco advertising in school buildings, on school grounds, on school buses or other vehicles used to transport students, in school publications, and through sponsorship of school events; and prohibited students from wearing tobacco brand-name apparel or carrying merchandise with tobacco company names, logos, or cartoon characters:** from 68.8% to 91.6% across states (median: 84.4%) and from 52.2% to 91.0% across cities (median: 79.2%) (Figure 6).

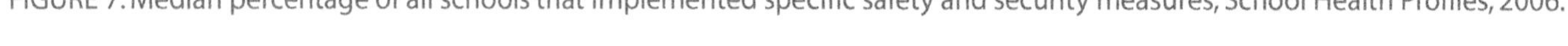

FIGURE 7. Median percentage of all schools that implemented specific safety and security measures, School Health Profiles, 2006.

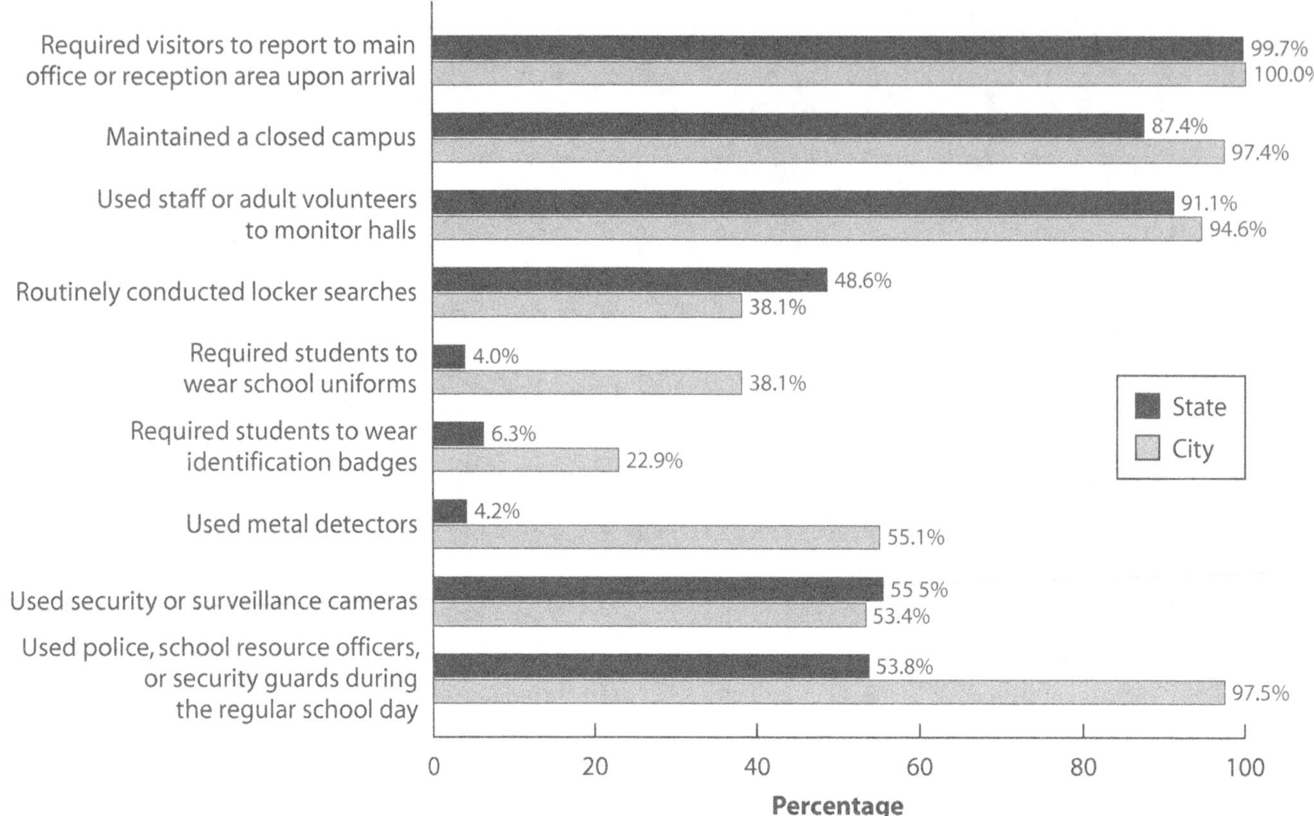

The percentage of all schools that provided referrals to tobacco cessation programs for faculty and staff ranged from 9.9% to 40.4% across states (median: 22.0%) and from 11.3% to 42.7% across cities (median: 20.7%) (Table 34). The percentage of all schools that provided referrals to tobacco cessation programs for students ranged from 17.8% to 81.2% across states (median: 47.9%) and from 19.8% to 96.4% across cities (median: 53.5%) (Table 34).

The percentage of all schools that posted signs marking a tobacco-free school zone, that is, a specified distance from school grounds where tobacco use is not allowed, ranged from 38.0% to 93.2% across states (median: 67.5%) and from 28.4% to 88.2% across cities (median: 80.6%) (Table 34a, b; Figure 6).

Violence Prevention

Schools implement measures to ensure the safety and security of students, staff, and visitors. The percentage of all schools that implemented specific safety and security measures ranged as follows (Table 35a, b; Figure 7):

- **Required visitors to report to the main office or reception area upon arrival:** from 92.3% to 100.0% across states (median: 99.7%) and from 98.9% to 100.0% across cities (median: 100.0%).

- **Maintained a "closed campus" where students are not allowed to leave school during the school day, including during lunchtime:** from 40.8% to 98.4% across states (median: 87.4%) and from 77.9% to 100.0% across cities (median: 97.4%).

- **Used staff or adult volunteers to monitor school halls during and between classes:** from 73.9% to 96.5% across states (median: 91.1%) and from 87.4% to 97.7% across cities (median: 94.6%).

- **Routinely conducted locker searches:** from 2.3% to 66.6% across states (median: 48.6%) and from 7.7% to 71.3% across cities (median: 38.1%).

- **Required students to wear school uniforms:** from 0.0% to 32.2% across states (median: 4.0%) and from 0.0% to 100.0% across cities (median: 38.1%).

- **Required students to wear identification badges:** from 0.7% to 42.8% across states (median: 6.3%) and from 3.2% to 98.0% across cities (median: 22.9%).

- **Used metal detectors, including wands:** from 0.0% to 37.6% across states (median: 4.2%) and from 1.8% to 95.3% across cities (median: 55.1%).

- **Used security or surveillance cameras, either inside or outside the school building:** from 20.5% to 85.3% across states (median: 55.5%) and from 6.2% to 100.0% across cities (median: 53.4%).

- **Use police, school resource officers, or security guards during the regular school day:** from 14.9% to 90.1% across states (median: 53.8%) and from 81.8% to 100.0% across cities (median: 97.5%).

The percentage of all schools that had or participated in specific violence prevention programs ranged as follows (Table 36):

- **A peer mediation program:** from 15.8% to 78.8% across states (median: 39.8%) and from 42.0% to 93.8% across cities (median: 70.0%).

- **A safe-passages to school program:** from 1.5% to 20.8% across states (median: 5.8%) and from 6.5% to 60.0% across cities (median: 24.9%).

- **A program to prevent gang violence:** from 8.0% to 55.7% across states (median: 23.9%) and from 42.1% to 89.7% across cities (median: 58.1%).

- **A program to prevent bullying:** from 30.8% to 83.6% across states (median: 65.1%) and from 45.3% to 96.9% across cities (median: 75.6%).

The percentage of all schools that had a comprehensive plan to address crisis preparedness, response, and recovery in the event of a natural disaster or other emergency or crisis situation ranged from 87.1% to 100.0% across states (median: 97.6%) and from 96.0% to 100.0% across cities (median: 100.0%) (Table 36).

HEALTH SERVICES

Schools can support student success by providing health services to students. The percentage of all schools that had a nurse who provided standard health services to students ranged from 28.9% to 100.0% across states (median: 90.6%) and from 16.0% to 100.0% across cities (median: 97.8%) (Table 37).

The percentage of all schools where a student would ever be permitted to carry and self-administer specific medications ranged as follows (Table 37):

- **Prescription quick-relief inhaler:** from 51.4% to 95.1% across states (median: 76.0%) and from 43.2% to 79.5% across cities (median: 66.8%).

- **Epinephrine auto-injector (e.g., EpiPen®):** from 23.9% to 64.1% across states (median: 45.3%) and from 8.3% to 67.7% across cities (30.7%).

- **Insulin or other injected medications:** from 10.5% to 64.4% across states (median: 31.0%) and from 2.1% to 41.6% across cities (median: 18.4%).

- **Any other prescribed medications:** from 2.6% to 45.2% across states (median: 11.1%) and from 1.7% to 34.3% across cities (median: 13.7%).

- **Any over-the-counter medications:** from 3.1% to 59.3% across states (median: 13.5%) and from 2.5% to 31.4% across cities (median: 12.2%).

The percentage of all schools that provided specific health services to students ranged as follows (Table 38):

- **Identification or school-based management of chronic health conditions, such as asthma or diabetes:** from 38.9% to 95.5% across states (median: 74.4%) and from 38.8% to 94.5% across cities (median: 79.4%).

- **Identification or school-based management of acute illnesses:** from 34.3% to 87.8% across states (median: 67.2%) and from 32.9% to 87.8% across cities (median: 68.0%).

- **Asthma Action Plan (or Individualized Health Plan) for all students with asthma:** from 22.8% to 86.8% across states (median: 65.4%) and from 19.7% to 86.9% across cities (median: 69.2%).

- **Immunizations:** from 32.1% to 80.7% across states (median: 49.9%) and from 36.1% to 76.8% across cities (median: 60.9%).

- **Assistance with enrolling in Medicaid or SCHIP (State Children's Health Insurance Program):** from 37.0% to 86.4% across states (median: 53.6%) and from 29.4% to 85.8% across cities (median: 59.2%).

POLICIES RELATED TO HIV INFECTION AND AIDS

School policies can provide critical support for HIV-infected students and staff. The percentage of all schools with a policy on students and/or staff who have HIV infection or AIDS ranged from 27.0% to 89.5% across states (median: 51.6%) and from 28.1% to 100.0% across cities (median: 46.8%) (Table 39). Among those schools that had a policy, the percentage whose policy addressed specific issues for students and/or staff with HIV infection or AIDS ranged as follows (Table 39a, b; Figure 8):

- **Attendance at school of students with HIV infection:** from 85.2% to 100.0% across states (median: 93.5%) and from 65.4% to 100.0% across cities (median: 91.0%).

- **Procedures to protect HIV-infected students and staff from discrimination:** from 93.3% to 100.0% across states (median: 97.3%) and from 93.0% to 100.0% across cities (median: 100.0%).

- **Maintenance of confidentiality of HIV-infected students and staff:** from 92.7% to 100.0% across states (median: 99.1%) and from 93.0% to 100.0% across cities (median: 100.0%).

- **Work site safety:** from 93.6% to 100.0% across states (median: 98.1%) and from 75.7% to 100.0% across cities (median: 100.0%).

- **Confidential counseling for HIV-infected students:** from 68.9% to 91.0% across states (median: 79.0%) and from 69.2% to 96.2% across cities (median: 89.2%).

- **Communication of the policy to students, school staff, and parents:** from 77.3% to 97.4% across states (median: 88.5%) and from 78.3% to 100.0% across cities (median: 90.1%).

FIGURE 8. Among schools with a policy on students or staff with HIV* infection or AIDS,† the median percentage whose policy addressed specific issues, School Health Profiles, 2006.

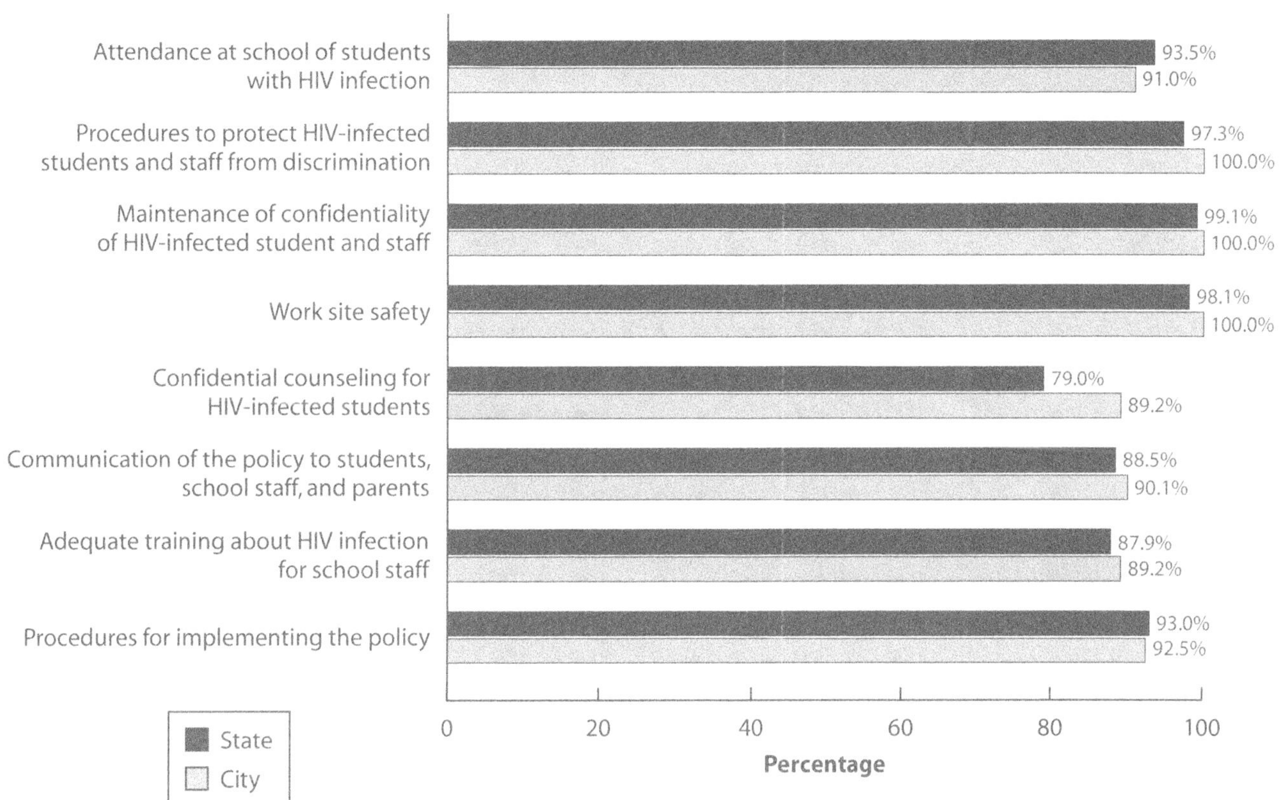

* Human immunodeficiency virus.
† Acquired immunodeficiency syndrome.

- **Adequate training about HIV infection for school staff:** from 67.2% to 95.5% across states (median: 87.9%) and from 55.1% to 100.0% across cities (median: 89.2%).

- **Procedures for implementing the policy:** from 84.7% to 98.0% across states (median: 93.0%) and from 78.7% to 100.0% across cities (median: 92.5%).

FAMILY AND COMMUNITY INVOLVEMENT

Partnerships between schools, families, and community members are important elements of a school health program. The percentage of all schools that had one or more than one group (e.g., a school health council, committee, or team) that offered guidance on the development of policies or coordinated activities on health topics ranged from 34.7% to 73.9% across states (median: 54.9%) and from 24.1% to 79.0% across cities (median: 48.4%) (Table 40).

The percentage of all schools that engaged parents and families in specific health education activities during the 2005–2006 school year ranged as follows (Table 40):

- **Provided families with information on school health education:** from 47.6% to 82.7% across states (median: 66.1%) and from 53.7% to 97.4% across cities (median: 69.3%).

- **Met with a parents' organization (e.g., the PTA) to discuss school health education:** from 10.5% to 32.8% across states (median: 22.3%) and from 18.8% to 63.3% across cities (median: 32.2%).

- **Invited family members to attend health education classes:** from 21.0% to 45.6% across states (median: 32.4%) and from 18.8% to 75.4% across cities (median: 41.8%).

The percentage of all schools that asked students to participate in health-related community activities as part of a required health education course during the 2005–2006 school year ranged as follows (Table 41):

- **Performed volunteer work at a hospital, a local health department, or any other local organization that addresses health issues:** from 6.2% to 24.8% across states (median: 13.0%) and from 0.0% to 36.9% across cities (median: 15.5%).

- **Participated in or attended a community health fair:** from 9.0% to 35.6% across states (median: 22.0%) and from 0.0% to 55.6% across cities (median: 23.9%).

- **Gathered information about health services that are available in the community, such as health screenings:** from 20.1% to 66.4% across states (median: 40.0%) and from 0.0% to 62.1% across cities (median: 36.8%).

- **Visited a store to compare prices of health products:** from 5.6% to 38.5% across states (median: 23.5%) and from 0.0% to 48.8% across cities (median: 22.4%).

- **Identified potential injury sites at school, home, or in the community:** from 22.4% to 70.0% across states (median: 48.5%) and from 0.0% to 70.0% across cities (median: 35.2%).

- **Identified advertising in the community designed to influence health behaviors:** from 28.2% to 79.6% across states (median: 61.4%) and from 0.0% to 88.2% across cities (median: 51.1%).

- **Advocated for a health-related issue:** from 23.1% to 82.2% across states (median: 44.6%) and from 0.0% to 59.7% across cities (median: 40.6%).

- **Completed homework or projects that involved family members:** from 34.1% to 90.2% across states (median: 71.1%) and from 0.0% to 94.5% across cities (median: 47.9%).

TRENDS

The Profiles were first conducted in 1996 and are repeated biennially. Although the questionnaires are modified each year, some questions remain constant, which allows investigators to analyze changes over time. **Long-term trends** compare median percentages calculated across all states or cities between the **1996**[67] and **2006** Profiles. **Short-term trends** compare median percentages between the **2004**[68] and **2006** Profiles.

LONG-TERM TRENDS

Significant improvements in school health practices and policies were detected between 1996 and 2006 in the following areas:

- Across **states**, the median percentage of all schools in which health education staff worked on health education activities with physical education staff, school health services staff, and nutrition or food service staff increased from 69.2% to 76.7%, from 44.3% to 66.4%, and from 18.2% to 37.9%, respectively.

- Across **states**, increases were found in the median percentage of all schools in which the lead health education teacher received staff development during the two years preceding the survey on alcohol-use or other drug-use prevention (from 40.3% to 50.4%), consumer health (from 9.3% to 22.2%), CPR (from 50.7% to 67.0%), dental and oral health (from 5.9% to 12.3%), emotional and mental health (from 21.4% to 35.6%), environmental health (from 8.8% to 14.2%), first aid (from 40.3% to 56.7%), growth and development (from 16.1% to 25.7%), injury prevention and safety (from 23.9% to 39.9%), nutrition and dietary behavior (from 26.9% to 35.4%), physical activity and fitness (from 31.9% to 48.3%), suicide prevention (from 15.6% to 25.5%), tobacco-use prevention (from 21.3% to 34.6%), and violence prevention (from 41.8% to 52.3%).

- Across **states**, increases were found in the median percentage of all schools in which the lead health education teacher wanted to receive staff development on alcohol-use or other drug-use prevention (from 53.5% to 72.5%), consumer health (from 33.0% to 49.4%), CPR (from 39.6% to 64.4%), dental and oral health (from 18.7% to 42.5%), emotional and mental health (from 53.5% to 67.4%), environmental health (from 38.6% to 52.5%), first aid (from 40.5% to 65.1%), growth and development (from 32.5% to 55.9%), HIV prevention (from 53.8% to 63.5%), human sexuality (from 50.6% to 57.3%), injury prevention and safety (from 34.4% to 59.6%), nutrition and dietary behavior (from 47.4% to 73.2%), physical activity and fitness (from 38.6% to 67.8%), pregnancy prevention (from 47.4% to 57.9%), STD prevention (from 55.0% to 62.8%), suicide prevention (from 68.3% to 72.3%), tobacco-use prevention (from 46.0% to 63.5%), and violence prevention (from 62.4% to 76.3%).

- Across **cities**, increases were found in the median percentage of all schools in which the lead health education teacher wanted to receive staff development on alcohol-use or other drug-use prevention (from 62.1% to 75.4%), dental and oral health (from 35.9% to 52.4%), emotional and mental health (from 65.6% to 77.7%), first aid (from 58.2% to 73.6%), growth and development (from 41.0% to 64.9%), HIV prevention (from 56.1% to 70.1%), human sexuality (from 46.2% to 69.1%), injury prevention and safety (from 43.2% to 64.3%), nutrition and dietary behavior (from 54.9% to 76.3%), physical activity and fitness (from 45.8% to 67.3%), pregnancy prevention (from 46.8% to 67.1%), STD prevention (from 52.7% to 70.0%), and tobacco-use prevention (from 47.1% to 66.0%).

- Across **states**, among schools that had adopted a policy on students and/or staff who have HIV infection or AIDS, increases were found in the median percentage of schools that had a policy that addressed the following issues for students and staff: procedures to protect HIV-infected students and staff from discrimination (from 90.4% to 97.3%); maintenance of confidentiality of HIV-infected students and staff (from 94.9% to 99.1%); work site safety (from 92.7% to 98.1%); communication of the policy to students, school staff, and parents (from 75.7% to 88.5%); and procedures for implementing the policy (from 86.2% to 93.0%).

- Across **cities**, the median percentage of all schools that had one or more than one group (e.g., a school health council, committee, or team) that offered guidance on the development of policies or coordinated activities on health topics increased from 18.7% to 48.4%.

Significant deteriorations in school health practices and policies were detected between 1996 and 2006 in the following areas:

- Across **states and cities**, the median percentage of all schools requiring teachers to use any state-developed, district-developed, or school-developed curriculum in a required health education course decreased from 84.5% to 75.3% and from 96.8% to 48.9%, respectively.

- Across **states**, the median percentage of all schools that tried to increase student knowledge on CPR in a required health education course decreased from 65.3% to 53.4%.

- Across **cities**, decreases were found in the median percentage of all schools that tried to increase student knowledge in a required health education course on alcohol-use or other drug-use prevention (from 96.6% to 57.6%), dental and oral health (from 75.0% to 41.3%), environmental health (from 71.8% to 47.2%), STD prevention (from 94.5% to 57.2%), and violence prevention (from 90.3% to 57.2%)

- Across **states**, the median percentage of all schools that tried to improve student decision-making skills in a required health education course decreased from 87.9% to 77.9%.

- Across **cities**, decreases were found in the median percentage of all schools that tried to improve student skills in a required health education course in communication (from 88.4% to 54.4%) and decision making (from 93.0% to 57.2%).

- Across **states**, decreases were found in the median percentage of all schools that taught in a required health education course abstinence as the most effective method to avoid pregnancy, HIV, and STDs (from 88.9% to 78.0%); how HIV is transmitted (from 91.9% to 78.7%); how HIV affects the human body (from 91.3% to 77.8%); condom efficacy (from 67.0% to 56.0%); influence of alcohol and other drugs on HIV-related risk behaviors (from 87.5% to 77.0%); social or cultural influences on sexual behavior (from 75.2% to 65.4%); and how to correctly use a condom (from 41.5% to 24.3%).

- Across **cities**, decreases were found in the median percentage of all schools that taught in a required health education course how HIV is transmitted (from 96.8% to 55.7%); how HIV affects the human body (from 94.8% to 55.7%); condom efficacy (from 75.9% to 53.0%); social or cultural influences on sexual behavior (from 85.6% to 49.4%); how to find valid information or services related to HIV or HIV testing (from 82.8% to 52.9%); how to correctly use a condom (from 67.4% to 34.2%); and compassion for persons living with HIV or AIDS (from 87.0% to 52.4%).

- Across **states and cities**, the median percentage of all schools in which the lead health education teacher had experience teaching health education classes or topics for 15 years or more decreased from 54.1% to 37.9% and from 67.3% to 36.0%, respectively.

- Across **states**, the median percentage of all schools in which the lead health education teacher received staff development during the 2 years preceding the survey on HIV prevention decreased from 51.4% to 43.7%.

- Across **states and cities**, the median percentage of all schools that had adopted a policy on students and/or staff who have HIV infection or AIDS decreased from 69.5% to 51.6% and from 82.5% to 46.8%, respectively.

SHORT-TERM TRENDS

Significant improvements in school health practices and policies were detected between 2004 and 2006 in the following areas:

- Across **states**, the median percentage of all schools that taught about using salt and sodium in moderation in a required health education course increased from 64.9% to 79.3%.

- Across **states**, the median percentage of all schools in which health education staff worked on health education activities with nutrition or food service staff increased from 23.4% to 37.9%.

- Across **states**, increases were found in the median percentage of all schools in which the lead health education teacher received staff development during the two years preceding the survey on consumer health (from 15.1% to 22.2%).

- Across **states**, increases were found in the median percentage of all schools in which the lead health education teacher wanted to receive staff development on CPR (from 58.0% to 64.4%), dental and oral health (from 33.7% to 42.5%), first aid (from 58.4% to 65.1%), growth and development (from 47.1% to 55.9%), immunizations (from 38.7% to 45.1%), injury prevention and safety (from 43.9% to 59.6%), nutrition and dietary behavior (from 64.8% to 73.2%), physical activity and fitness (from 57.6% to 67.8%), and sun safety or skin cancer prevention (from 48.2% to 55.9%).

- Across **states**, the median percentage of all schools that had a policy stating that if food is served at student parties, after-school or extended day programs, or concession stands, fruits and vegetables would be among the foods offered increased from 9.7% to 17.8%.

- Across **states**, the median percentage of all schools that allowed students to purchase snack foods or beverages from vending machines or at a school store, canteen, or snack bar decreased from 89.5% to 83.3%.

- Across **states**, decreases were found in the median percentage of all schools that allowed students to purchase from vending machines or at the school store, canteen, or snack bar chocolate candy (from 52.6% to 40.3%), other kinds of candy (from 55.2% to 43.6%), and salty snacks that are not low in fat (from 63.7% to 47.4%).

- Across **states**, the median percentage of all schools that allowed students to purchase candy; snacks that are not low in fat; soda pop, sports drinks, or fruit drinks that are not 100% juice; or 2% or whole milk during school lunch periods decreased from 51.7% to 34.9%.

Significant deteriorations in school health practices and policies were detected between 2004 and 2006 in the following areas:

- Across **states** and **cities**, the median percentage of all schools requiring teachers to use any state-developed, district-developed, or school-developed curriculum in a required health education course decreased from 96.8% to 75.3% and from 100.0% to 48.9%, respectively.

- Across **states**, among schools that required a physical education course for students in any of grades 6 through 12, the median percentage that allowed students to be exempted from taking a required physical education course for enrollment in other courses increased from 6.9% to 15.2%.

- Across **states** and **cities**, the median percentage of all schools that had adopted a policy on students and/or staff who have HIV infection or AIDS decreased from 59.4% to 51.6% and from 65.3% to 46.8%, respectively.

- Across **cities**, the median percentage of all schools that had one or more than one group (e.g., a school health council, committee, or team) that offered guidance on the development of policies or coordinated activities on health topics decreased from 72.3% to 48.4%.

DISCUSSION

Coordinated school health programs (CSHPs) help students develop and improve health-related knowledge, attitudes, and skills. In addition, these programs can help improve health behaviors, health outcomes, educational outcomes, and social outcomes among adolescents and young adults.[69] School Health Profiles provides information to help assess some aspects of five of the eight components of CSHPs. Long-term and short-term trends in Profiles data illustrate how school health policies and programs have evolved over time to meet the needs of students and demonstrate areas for improvement.

By providing school-level data that is representative of each participating state and large urban school district, Profiles complements the School Health Policies and Programs Study (SHPPS). SHPPS was conducted most recently in 2006, and provides nationally representative data on school health policies and programs related to all eight components of CSHPs.[70]

The *National Health Education Standards*, the Institute of Medicine, and the *Healthy People 2010* objectives all identify health education as important to help keep America's youth healthy.[5,9,10] Profiles measures many characteristics of health education. For example, across states, the median percentage of all schools that taught a required health education course in a particular grade decreased from 51.3% in grade 6 to 14.7% in grade 12. These results are of concern because as a student's grade increases, the prevalence of many health risk behaviors also increases,[55] creating an even greater need for required health education in higher grades.

Healthy People 2010[10] Objective 7-2 specifies that the following topics be addressed in health education: unintentional injuries; violence; suicide; tobacco use and addiction; alcohol and other drug use; unintended pregnancy, HIV/AIDS, and STD infections; unhealthy dietary patterns; inadequate physical activity; and environmental health. Across states, a median of more than 75% of all middle schools and high schools tried to increase student knowledge on tobacco-use prevention; alcohol-use or other drug-use prevention; HIV, STD, and pregnancy prevention; nutrition and dietary behavior; and physical activity and fitness. Across cities, however, the median percentage of all middle and high schools that tried to increase student knowledge did not exceed 60% for any topic.

In addition, since 1996, a significant decrease occurred in the median percentage of all middle and high schools across states that taught about abstinence as the most effective method to avoid pregnancy, HIV, and STDs; how HIV is transmitted; how HIV affects the human body; condom efficacy; influence of alcohol and other drugs on HIV-related risk behaviors; social or cultural influences on sexual behavior; and how to correctly use a condom. For cities, a significant decrease occurred in the median percentage of all middle and high schools that taught about alcohol-use or other drug-use prevention, dental and oral health, environmental health, STD prevention, and violence prevention. Concurrently, a significant decrease occurred in the median percentage of all middle schools and high schools across cities that taught how HIV is transmitted; how HIV affects the human body; condom efficacy; social or cultural influences on sexual behavior; how to find valid information or services related to HIV or HIV testing; how to correctly use a condom; and compassion for persons living with HIV or AIDS.

These results are of concern, in general, because schools need to ensure that health education topics address the priority health problems identified by the *Healthy People 2010*[10] objectives, and specifically, because the impact of the HIV epidemic is continuing to grow in many communities.

The *National Health Education Standards* identify particular student skills such as goal setting, decision making, communication, and stress management that are important for enhancing health.[9] More than 70% of all middle schools and high schools across states tried to improve student skills in finding valid health information, products, and services. Middle schools and high schools also tried to reduce the influence of media on personal health and wellness; improve communication, decision-making, goal-setting, and conflict resolution skills; and promote attitudes to resist peer pressure for engaging in unhealthy behaviors.

Since 1996, across states, a significant decrease occurred in the median percentage of all middle schools and high schools that tried to improve student skills in decision making. During the same period, across cities, a significant decrease also occurred in the median percentage of all middle schools and high schools that tried to improve student skills in communication and decision making.

An important component of effective health education is that an individual is appointed to coordinate it.[5] More than 90% of all middle and high schools across states and cities have a health education coordinator. It is also important that health education teachers be trained in health education. In 2006, professional preparation of the lead health education teacher varied greatly across states and cities. The median percentage of all middle and high school lead health education teachers who had professional preparation in health education was 4.7% across states and 8.0% across cities. The median percentage of all health education teachers who had professional preparation in health and physical education combined was 45.5% across states and 26.4% across cities.

Coordination of health education activities with other components of the school health program helps ensure that health issues are consistently addressed and reinforced within schools. The median percentage of all middle and high schools across states and cities that worked on health education activities with physical education, health services, and mental health or social services staff was more than 50%. Since 1996, across states, a significant increase occurred in the median percentage of all middle schools and high schools that worked on health education activities with physical education, school health services, and nutrition or food service staff. Coordination between health education and other school staff may improve the implementation of health education activities.

CDC guidelines, *Healthy People 2010* objectives, and NASPE standards recommend required daily physical education to promote active, productive, and healthy lifestyles among youth.[10,27,29] In 2006, the median percentage of all schools across states and cities that required physical education for students in any of grades 6 through 12 was more than 90%. Across states and cities, however, the median percentage of all schools that taught a required PE course in a particular grade decreased as grade level increased. This is a cause for concern because as students' grade increases, the amount of physical activity they engage in tends to decrease.[55]

School health services help students appraise, protect, and improve their health. One major aspect of health services is helping students with asthma manage their illness. In 2006, more than 65% of all schools across states and cities provided all students having asthma with an Asthma Action Plan, permitted students to carry and self-administer a prescription quick-relief inhaler, and provided identification or school-based management of chronic health conditions, such as asthma.

Across states and cities, the median percentage of all schools in which the lead health education teacher received staff development during the two years preceding the survey on asthma awareness was 19.2% and 33.8%, respectively. However, the median percentage of all schools in which the lead health education teacher wanted to receive staff development on asthma awareness was 56.5% across states and 66.2% across cities.

The Child Nutrition and WIC Reauthorization Act of 2004 requires school districts that participate in the National School Lunch Program or the School Breakfast Program to develop a local wellness policy that must address nutrition education and provide nutrition guidelines for all foods available on school campuses.[46] The Institute of Medicine report, *Nutrition Standards for Foods in Schools: Leading the Way Toward Healthier Youth*[47] provides specific recommendations for foods and beverages sold outside of the school meal programs that schools, districts, and states should consider when developing or strengthening policies related to nutrition in schools.

Across states a significant increase was noted between 2004 and 2006 in the median percentage of all schools that had a policy stating that if food is served at student parties, at after-school or extended-day programs, or at concession stands, then fruits and vegetables would be among the foods offered. During this same period, a significant decrease was detected in the median percentage of all schools across states that allowed students to purchase chocolate candy, other kinds of candy, and salty snacks that are not low in fat from vending machines or at the school store, canteen, or snack bar. In addition, a decrease was noted between 2004 and 2006 in the median percentage of all schools across states that allowed students to purchase candy; snacks that are not low in fat; soda pop, sports drinks, fruit drinks that are not 100% juice; or 2% or whole milk during school lunch periods.

The No Child Left Behind Act of 2001 reauthorized the Pro-Children Act of 1994, which prohibits smoking in any indoor facility that receives federal funds and provides routine or regular education, day care, health care, early childhood development, or library services to children.[52,71] The Pro-Children Act is generally limited to indoor facilities in an attempt to protect children from secondhand smoke. CDC's *Guidelines for School Health Programs to Prevent Tobacco Use and Addiction* identified key elements of a school tobacco-use prevention policy.[50] Such a policy should prohibit tobacco use by students, faculty, staff, and visitors on school property; in all school vehicles; and at school-sponsored functions away from school property. Across states and cities, the median percentage of all schools that prohibited all tobacco use in all locations was 53.8% and 56.0%, respectively. More schools should adopt and enforce components of a tobacco-use prevention policy to meet the *Healthy People 2010* objective of 100% tobacco-free school environments.[10] Another strategy identified in CDC's guidelines to aid schools in preventing tobacco use among youth is the prohibition of tobacco advertising in school buildings, on school property, and in school publications. In 2006, more than 90% of all schools across states and cities prohibited tobacco advertising in school buildings, on school grounds, on all school vehicles, and in school publications. In addition, more than 90% of all schools across states and cities prohibited tobacco advertising through sponsorship of school events and prohibited students from wearing tobacco brand-name apparel or carrying merchandise with tobacco company names, logos, or cartoon characters on it.

The No Child Left Behind Act of 2001 also authorized schools to use federal funds for programs to prevent violence in and around schools.[52] In 2006, the median percentage of all schools that used metal detectors and had uniformed police, undercover police, or security guards during the regular school day varied greatly between states and cities.

School policies should address the needs of students and staff with HIV infection and AIDS. Across states and cities, a decrease occurred from 1996 to 2006 in the median percentage of all schools that had adopted a policy on students and/or staff who have HIV infection or AIDS. However, across states, among schools that had adopted a policy, increases were found in the median percentage of schools that had a policy that addressed several key issues, including procedures to protect HIV-infected students and staff from discrimination; maintenance of confidentiality of HIV-infected students and staff; workplace safety; communication of the HIV policy to students, school staff, and parents; and procedures for implementing the policy.

Collaboration between schools and families is essential to the success of CSHPs. More than 65% of all schools across states and cities provided information on school health education to families. However, less than 35% of schools met with a parents' organization, such as the PTA, to discuss school health education, or invited family members to attend health education classes.

Several limitations should be noted. The data presented in this report apply only to public middle schools and high schools and are limited to these school populations. Because the data were combined across both school levels, program and policy differences between the two levels may be masked. Second, the data are self-reported by school principals and lead health education teachers and may be subject to bias. Finally, the Profiles data do not provide an in-depth assessment of all elements of a CSHP.[2]

State and local education and health agencies use Profiles data to advocate for health and physical education programs, promote curricula or program modifications, support school health legislation, and identify staff development needs. For example, the Rhode Island Departments of Education and Health used Profiles data to plan and prioritize technical assistance activities with school districts to support health and physical education curriculum development. In addition, both agencies used data from Profiles in support of a legislative bill to require that only healthier snacks and beverages be sold or distributed in schools. The State of Alaska Department of Education and Early Development used 2006 Profiles data to identify the staff development needs of health education and physical education teachers. In response, the department conducted statewide training on several health topics. The Montana Office of Public Instruction used Profiles data to support several legislative bills and recommendations to increase the amount of time spent by students in physical education classes. In addition, Montana schools used Profiles data in their School Wellness policy development and implementation efforts.

Profiles data help state and local education and health agencies promote program strengths and advocate for resources to address weaknesses. Numerous resources exist to help states and districts address weaknesses identified through their Profiles data. For example, for states and districts needing to improve their policies, *The Food-Safe Schools Action Guide* helps schools identify gaps in food safety and develop policies to prevent foodborne illness.[72] *Fit, Healthy, and Ready to Learn* is another guide to help schools develop policies to address physical activity, healthy eating, tobacco-use prevention, asthma control, and a healthy school environment.[73,74] The guide includes information on the policy development process, general school health policies, and examples of specific policies for all topic areas. CDC's School Health Index (SHI) is a tool to help schools identify strengths and weakness of their health and safety policies and practices through a self-assessment process and to develop an action plan for improvement. The process engages teachers, parents, students, and the community to help promote positive health behaviors.[75] Finally, *Making it Happen: School Nutrition Success Stories* describes how schools across the United States improved the types of foods and beverages sold and offered outside of the USDA school meal program to provide more healthy choices for students.[76]

REFERENCES

1. Snyder T, Dillow S, Hoffman C. *Digest of Educational Statistics 2006*. Washington, DC: U.S. Department of Education, National Center for Education Statistics; 2007. Publication No. NCES 2007017.

2. Allensworth D, Kolbe L. The comprehensive school health program: exploring an expanded concept. *Journal of School Health* 1987;57(10):409–412.

3. SAS Institute, Inc. SAS,® version 9.1 [Software and documentation]. Research Triangle Park, NC: Research Triangle Institute; 2004.

4. Armitage P, Berry G. *Statistical Methods in Medical Research*. 3rd edition. Cambridge, MA: Blackwell Scientific Publications, Inc.; 1994:448–468.

5. Institute of Medicine. *School and Health: Our Nation's Investment*. Washington, DC: National Academy Press; 1997.

6. Lohrmann D, Wooley S. Comprehensive school health education. In: Marx E, Wooley S, eds., with Northrop D. *Health is Academic: A Guide to School Health Programs*. New York: Teachers College Press; 1998:43–66.

7. McKenzie F, Richmond J. Linking health and learning: an overview of coordinated school health. In: Marx E, Wooley S, eds., with Northrop D. *Health Is Academic: A Guide to School Health Programs*. New York: Teachers College Press; 1998:1–14.

8. Joint Committee on National Health Education Standards. *National Health Education Standards: Achieving Health Literacy*. Atlanta: American Cancer Society; 1995.

9. Joint Committee on National Health Education Standards. *National Health Education Standards: Achieving Excellence*. Atlanta: American Cancer Society; 2007.

10. U.S. Department of Health and Human Services. *Healthy People 2010*. 2nd ed. with *Understanding and Improving Health and Objectives for Improving Health*, 2 vols. Washington, DC: U.S. Department of Health and Human Services; 2000.

11. American Cancer Society. *Improving School Health: A Guide to the Role of School Health Coordinator*. Atlanta: American Cancer Society; 1999.

12. Palmer J. Planning wheels turn curriculum around. *Educational Leader* 1991;49:57–60.

13. Public Education Network. *Teacher Professional Development: A Primer for Parents and Community Members*. Washington, D.C.: Public Education Network; 2004.

14. Lavin A. Comprehensive school health education: barriers and opportunities. *Journal of School Health* 1993;63(1):24–7.

15. Jones SE, Brener ND, McManus T. The relationship between staff development and health instruction in schools in the United States. *American Journal of Health Education* 2004;35:2–10.

16. Ross J, Luepker R, Nelson G, Saavedra P, Hubbard B. Teenage health teaching modules: impact of teacher training on implementation and student outcomes. *Journal of School Health* 1991;61(1):31–34.

17. U.S. Department of Health and Human Services. *The Surgeon General's Call to Action to Prevent and Decrease Overweight and Obesity*. Rockville, MD: U.S. Department of Health and Human Services, Public Health Service, Office of the Surgeon General; 2001.

18. Lichtenstein A, Appel L, Brands M, et al. Diet and lifestyle recommendations revision 2006: a scientific statement from the American Heart Association nutrition committee. *Circulation* 2006;114(1):84–96.

19. Jemal A, Siegel R, Ward E, Murray T, Xu J, Thun M. Cancer statistics, 2007. *A Cancer Journal for Clinicians* 2007;57(1):43–66.

20. Centers for Disease Control and Prevention. *National Diabetes Fact Sheet: General Information and National Estimates on Diabetes in the United States, 2005*. Atlanta: U.S. Department of Health and Human Services, Centers for Disease Control and Prevention; 2005.

21. U.S. Department of Health and Human Services. *Physical Activity and Health: A Report of the Surgeon General*. Atlanta, GA: U.S. Department of Health and Human Services, Centers for Disease Control and Prevention, National Center for Chronic Disease Prevention and Health Promotion; 1996.

22. Ogden CL. Prevalence of overweight and obesity in the United States, 1999–2004. *JAMA* 2006;295(13):1549 –1555.

23. Caspersen CJ, Pereira MA, Curran KM. Changes in physical activity patterns in the United States, by sex and cross-sectional age. *Medicine and Science in Sports and Exercise* 2000;32(9):1601–1609.

24. Sallis JF. Age-related decline in physical activity: a synthesis of human and animal studies. *Medicine and Science in Sports and Exercise* 2000;32(9):1598–600.

25. Gordon-Larsen P, Nelson MC, Popkin BM. Longitudinal physical activity and sedentary behavior trends: adolescence to adulthood. *American Journal of Preventive Medicine* 2004;27(4):277–283.

26. Nelson MC, Neumark-Sztainer D, Hannan PJ, Sirard JR, Story M. Longitudinal and secular trends in physical activity and sedentary behavior during adolescence. *Pediatrics* 2006;118(6):1627–1634.

27. CDC. Guidelines for school and community programs to promote lifelong physical activity among young people. *Morbidity and Mortality Weekly Report* 1997;46(RR-6):1–36.

28. Task Force on Community Preventive Services. Recommendations to increase physical activity in communities. *American Journal of Preventive Medicine* 2002;22(4S):67–72.

29. National Association for Sport and Physical Education. *Moving into the Future: National Standards for Physical Education*. 2nd ed. Reston, VA: National Association for Sport and Physical Education; 2004.

30. American Academy of Pediatrics. *School Health: Policy and Practice*. Elk Grove Village, IL: American Academy of Pediatrics; 2004.

31. National Association of School Nurses. *School Health Nursing Services Role in Health Care: Role of the School Nurse*. Castle Rock, CO: National Association of School Nurses; 2002. Available at http://www.nasn.org/Default.aspx?tabid=279.

32. Centers for Disease Control and Prevention. Surveillance for asthma—United States, 1980–1999. *Morbidity and Mortality Weekly Report* 2002;51 (SS-1):1–13.

33. Centers for Disease Control and Prevention. *Asthma Prevalence, Health Care Use, and Mortality, 2002.* Hyattsville, MD: U.S. Department of Health and Human Services, National Center for Health Statistics; 2005. Available at http://www.cdc.gov/nchs/products/pubs/pubd/hestats/asthma/asthma.htm.

34. Lieu T, Lozano P, Finklestein J, et al. Racial/ethnic variation in asthma status and management practices among children in managed Medicaid. *Pediatrics* 2002;109(5):857–865.

35. American Lung Association. *Trends in Asthma Morbidity and Mortality*. New York: American Lung Association; 2007.

36. Centers for Disease Control and Prevention. Strategies for addressing asthma within a coordinated school health program. Atlanta: U.S. Department of Health and Human Services; 2002.

37. American Diabetes Association. Type 2 diabetes in children and adolescents. *Pediatrics* 2000;105:671–680.

38. Fagot-Campagna A, Narayan KMV, Impertatore G. Type 2 diabetes in children. *BMJ* 2001;322:377–378.

39. U.S. Department of Agriculture. *School Breakfast Program Participation and Meals Served*, 2007. Available at http://www.fns.usda.gov/pd/sbsummar.htm.

40. U.S. Department of Agriculture. *National School Lunch Program: foods sold in competition with USDA school meal programs: a report to Congress, 2001*. Washington, D.C.: U.S. Department of Agriculture; 2001. Available at http://www.fns.usda.gov/cnd/Lunch/CompetitiveFoods/report_congress.htm.

41. U.S. Department of Agriculture. *School meals: foods of minimal nutritional value*, 2003. Washington, D.C.: U.S. Department of Agriculture; 2003. Available at http://www.fns.usda.gov/cnd/menu/fmnv.htm.

42. Dietary Reference Intakes (DRIs): Recommended Intakes for Individuals. National Academies. Available at http://www.iom.edu/Object.File/Master/21/372/0.pdf.

43. Wright J, Wang C, Kennedy-Stephenson J, Ervin R. Dietary intake of ten key nutrients for public health, United States: 1999–2000. *Advance Data from Vital and Health Statistics* 2003;334.

44. Ervin R, Wang C, Wright J, Kennedy-Stephenson J. Dietary intake of ten key nutrients for public health, United States: 1999–2000. *Advance Data from Vital and Health Statistics* 2004;341.

45. Institute of Medicine. Dietary reference intakes for energy, carbohydrate, fiber, fat, fatty acids, cholesterol, protein, and amino acids. Washington, D.C.: National Academy Press; 2002.

46. Child Nutrition and Women, Infants, and Children Reauthorization Act of 2004, Pub. L. No. 108–265.

47. Institute of Medicine. *Nutrition Standards for Foods in Schools: Leading the Way Toward Healthier Youth.* Washington, D.C.: The National Academic Press; 2007.

48. Centers for Disease Control and Prevention. Annual smoking-attributable mortality, years of potential life lost, and economic costs — United States, 1997–2001. *Morbidity and Mortality Weekly Report* 2005;54(25):625–628.

49. Centers for Disease Control and Prevention. *Preventing Tobacco Use Among Young People: A Report of the Surgeon General.* Atlanta: U.S. Department of Health and Human Services, Public Health Service; 1994.

50. Centers for Disease Control and Prevention. Guidelines for school health programs to prevent tobacco use and addiction. *Morbidity and Mortality Weekly Report* 1994;43(RR-2):1–18.

51. Heron MP, Smith BL. Deaths: leading causes for 2003. *National Vital Statistics Report* 2007;55(10). Available at http://www.cdc.gov/nchs/data/nvsr/nvsr55/nvsr55_10.pdf.

52. No Child Left Behind Act of 2001, Pub. L. No. 107 110, §1061, 115 Stat. 2083 (2002).

53. Centers for Disease Control and Prevention. School health guidelines to prevent unintentional injury and violence. *Morbidity and Mortality Weekly Report* 2001;50(RR-22):1–73.

54. Centers for Disease Control and Prevention. *HIV/AIDS Surveillance in Adolescents*, Slide Series L265 (through 2005). Available at http://www.cdc.gov/hiv/topics/surveillance/resources/slides/adolescents/index.htm.

55. Centers for Disease Control and Prevention. Youth Risk Behavior Surveillance — United States, 2005. *Morbidity and Mortality Weekly Report* 2006;55(No. SS-5).

56. National Association of State Boards of Education. *Someone at School Has AIDS: A Comprehensive Guide to Education Policies Concerning HIV Infection.* Alexandria, VA: National Association of State Boards of Education; 1996.

57. Centers for Disease Control and Prevention. *Executive Summary—Improving the Health of Adolescents and Young Adults: A Guide for States and Communities*. Atlanta: Centers for Disease Control and Prevention; 2004.

58. Carlyon P, Carlyon W, McCarthy A. Family and community involvement in school health. In: Marx E, Wooley S, eds., with Northrop D. *Health is Academic: A Guide to School Health Programs*. New York: Teachers College Press; 1998:67–95.

59. Epstein JL. *School, Family, and Community Partnerships: Preparing Educators and Improving Schools*. Boulder, CO: Westview Press, 2001.

60. Golan M, Crow S. Targeting parents exclusively in the treatment of childhood obesity: long term results. *Obesity Research* 2004;2:357–361.

61. Lantz PM, Jacobson PD, Warner KE, Wasserman J, Pollack HA, Berson J, Ahlstrom A. Investing in youth tobacco control: a review of smoking prevention and control strategies. *Tobacco Control* 2000;9:47–63.

62. National Asthma Education and Prevention Program. Students with Chronic Illnesses: Guidance for Families, Schools and Students. National Heart, Lung, and Blood Institute, 2002. Available at http://www.nhlbi.nih.gov/health/public/lung/asthma/guidfam.htm.

63. Wheeler LS, Merkle SL, Gerald LB, Taggart VS. Managing asthma in schools: lessons learned and recommendations. *Journal of School Health* 2006;76(6):340–344.

64. Council of Chief State School Officers. Joint Work Group. Essential tips for successful collaboration. Washington, D.C.: Council of Chief State School Officers; 2004.

65. What Education Leaders Should Know About Forming Partnerships to Prevent Sexual-Risk Behaviors in School-Aged Youth. Washington, D.C.: Council of Chief State School Officers; 2005.

66. Kirby D, Laris BA, Rolleri L. Sex and HIV education programs for youth: their impact and important characteristics. Washington D.C.: Family Health International; 2006. Available at http://www.etr.org/recapp/programs/SexHIVedProgs.pdf.

67. Centers for Disease Control and Prevention. Surveillance for characteristics of health education among secondary schools—School Health Education Profiles, 1996. *Morbidity and Mortality Weekly Report* 1998;47(SS-4):1–31.

68. Grunbaum JA, Di Pietra J, McManus T, Hawkins J, Kann L. *School Health Profiles: Characteristics of Health Programs Among Secondary Schools (Profiles 2004)*. Atlanta: U.S. Department of Health and Human Services, Centers for Disease Control and Prevention; 2005.

69. Kolbe LJ. Education reform and the goals of modern school health programs. *The State Education Standard* 2002;3:4–11.

70. Kann L, Brener ND, Wechsler H. Overview and summary: School Health Policies and Programs Study 2006. *Journal of School Health* 2007;77:385–397.

71. Pro-Children Act of 1994, 20 U.S.D.S. §6081 *et seq*. (2001).

72. Centers for Disease Control and Prevention. Food-Safe Schools Action Guide. Available at http://www.cdc.gov/HealthyYouth/foodsafety/actionguide.htm.

73. Bogden JF, Vega-Matos CA. *Fit, Healthy, and Ready to Learn*. Alexandria, VA: National Association of State Boards of Education; 2000.

74. Wilson TK, Bogden JF. *Fit, Healthy, and Ready to Learn, Part III*. Alexandria, VA: National Association of State Boards of Education; 2005.

75. Centers for Disease Control and Prevention. School Health Index: A Self-Assessment and Planning Guide. Available at http://www.cdc.gov/healthyyouth/shi.

76. Food and Nutrition Service, U.S. Department of Agriculture; Centers for Disease Control and Prevention, U.S. Department of Health and Human Services; U.S. Department of Education. FNS-374, Making it Happen: School nutrition success stories. Available at http://www.cdc.gov/healthyyouth/nutrition/making-it-happen/index.htm.

TABLES

TABLE 1. Sample Sizes and Response Rates, Selected U.S. Sites: School Health Profiles, Principal and Lead Health Education Teacher Surveys, 2006

	Principal surveys		Teacher surveys	
Site	Sample size	Response rate (%)	Sample size	Response rate (%)
STATE SURVEYS				
Alabama	260	77	252	74
Alaska	223	76	206	71
Arizona	337	85	307	78
Arkansas	254	79	249	78
Connecticut	244	77	238	75
Delaware	68	91	68	91
Florida	299	72	298	71
Georgia	279	72	271	70
Hawaii	78	74	78	74
Idaho	213	89	201	84
Illinois	318	70	NA†	NA
Iowa	273	78	275	79
Kansas	253	78	243	75
Maine	277	85	255	78
Massachusetts	661	88	659	88
Michigan	346	86	323	80
Mississippi	180	76	173	73
Missouri	333	85	321	82
Montana	263	81	253	78
Nebraska	236	82	222	77
New Hampshire	182	85	165	77
New York*	367	79	356	77
North Carolina	299	71	299	71
North Dakota	166	76	168	77
Oregon	272	79	255	74
Pennsylvania	349	78	342	76
Rhode Island	88	77	88	77
South Carolina	248	78	245	77
South Dakota	206	72	202	71
Tennessee	318	80	303	77
Texas	362	71	358	71
Utah	209	82	182	71
Vermont	136	88	114	74
Virginia	280	74	277	74
Washington	269	71	NA	NA
West Virginia	196	86	196	86

TABLE 1. Sample Sizes and Response Rates, Selected U.S. Sites: School Health Profiles, Principal and Lead Health Education Teacher Surveys, 2006 *(continued)*

	Principal surveys		Teacher surveys	
Site	Sample size	Response rate (%)	Sample size	Response rate (%)
LOCAL SURVEYS				
Charlotte-Mecklenburg County	42	86	40	82
Chicago	234	77	212	70
Dallas	51	98	52	100
District of Columbia	31	72	32	74
Hillsborough County	55	83	58	88
Los Angeles	87	73	90	76
Memphis	58	85	56	82
Miami	90	93	83	86
Orange County	35	71	35	71
Philadelphia	106	73	104	71
San Diego	57	98	56	97
San Francisco	34	79	34	79

* Survey did not include schools from the New York City Department of Education.
† Data not available.

TABLE 2. Percentage of Schools That Required Health Education in Any of Grades 6–12, the Percentage That Required Students to Take Only One Course or Two or More Courses, and Among Schools That Required Health Education, the Percentage That Taught Required Health Education in a Combined Course or in Another Course and the Percentage That Required Students Who Fail a Required Health Education Course to Repeat It, Selected U.S. Sites: School Health Profiles, Principal Surveys, 2006

Site	Required health education	Required only one health education course	Required two or more health education courses	Taught required health education in a combined health education and physical education course*	Taught required health education in a course mainly about another subject*†	Required students who fail a required health education course to repeat it*
STATE SURVEYS						
Alabama	86.4	57.1	18.8	59.3	33.0	76.6
Alaska	82.2	35.5	44.4	64.3	25.5	85.1
Arizona	55.6	29.4	16.2	67.1	37.4	47.0
Arkansas	97.0	52.0	43.3	60.2	21.8	74.0
Connecticut	89.7	29.3	53.0	52.7	19.6	46.8
Delaware	95.3	37.9	50.8	81.1	9.8	52.6
Florida	70.8	42.9	19.0	65.3	33.6	68.6
Georgia	90.9	52.1	37.4	81.3	15.4	53.4
Hawaii	93.5	62.5	30.6	62.0	18.6	65.5
Idaho	98.1	55.3	42.3	50.2	8.1	56.5
Illinois	97.3	46.2	46.4	62.2	15.3	54.5
Iowa	76.1	33.0	37.4	40.8	31.7	56.0
Kansas	88.3	49.6	29.8	86.8	22.2	64.8
Maine	93.4	39.0	49.2	49.2	17.6	50.4
Massachusetts	85.6	28.9	52.0	54.0	10.2	39.2
Michigan	82.1	45.9	29.4	53.0	21.5	57.0
Mississippi	91.5	82.4	8.1	42.3	15.9	95.4
Missouri	88.4	43.3	42.9	66.0	17.7	57.3
Montana	98.6	15.5	79.3	93.9	24.5	63.5
Nebraska	93.5	39.3	50.1	77.4	25.4	57.2
New Hampshire	88.5	39.0	42.0	40.7	15.3	52.2
New York‡	99.4	39.5	59.9	32.8	10.6	58.0
North Carolina	95.2	42.5	46.4	93.7	15.0	51.7
North Dakota	92.9	26.4	63.6	64.0	24.7	58.9
Oregon	98.0	21.5	73.2	59.5	21.3	54.7
Pennsylvania	97.0	30.6	65.1	70.0	13.9	52.2
Rhode Island	97.7	16.2	74.6	81.2	7.6	41.8
South Carolina	85.5	42.0	34.7	73.4	26.4	35.0
South Dakota	71.3	23.2	41.8	80.4	21.1	38.8
Tennessee	77.6	42.7	24.1	87.4	30.0	59.0
Texas	81.0	62.0	14.6	51.4	19.6	74.2
Utah	97.7	64.9	31.8	41.0	10.5	49.3
Vermont	87.0	32.3	41.5	47.6	29.7	54.0
Virginia	91.4	12.5	68.4	98.0	10.5	48.3
Washington	92.7	43.5	43.0	68.0	27.7	57.6
West Virginia	98.9	38.6	58.6	47.6	7.2	46.3
State Median	**91.5**	**39.4**	**43.0**	**63.1**	**19.6**	**55.4**
State Range	**55.6 – 99.4**	**12.5 – 82.4**	**8.1 – 79.3**	**32.8 – 98.0**	**7.2 – 37.4**	**35.0 – 95.4**

TABLE 2. Percentage of Schools That Required Health Education in Any of Grades 6–12, the Percentage That Required Students to Take Only One Course or Two or More Courses, and Among Schools That Required Health Education, the Percentage That Taught Required Health Education in a Combined Course or in Another Course and the Percentage That Required Students Who Fail a Required Health Education Course to Repeat It, Selected U.S. Sites: School Health Profiles, Principal Surveys, 2006 *(continued)*

Site	Required health education	Required only one health education course	Required two or more health education courses	Taught required health education in a combined health education and physical education course*	Taught required health education in a course mainly about another subject*†	Required students who fail a required health education course to repeat it*
LOCAL SURVEYS						
Charlotte-Mecklenburg County	100.0	33.1	66.9	100.0	0.0	45.6
Chicago	76.6	33.2	20.2	88.7	45.2	35.1
Dallas	60.8	44.8	12.0	23.9	14.1	86.2
District of Columbia	97.0	29.0	54.4	96.9	14.3	66.6
Hillsborough County	56.0	44.2	7.5	49.5	42.1	64.3
Los Angeles	100.0	74.7	25.3	12.4	41.2	49.8
Memphis	85.6	55.5	25.4	95.2	3.4	57.4
Miami	59.2	46.3	10.3	77.6	36.6	77.1
Orange County	59.6	32.8	8.1	56.1	51.7	84.8
Philadelphia	88.7	50.0	35.2	92.6	19.5	35.1
San Diego§	100.0	0.0	0.0	59.2	90.9	0.0
San Francisco	91.3	45.5	11.5	46.6	54.4	60.2
Local Median	**87.2**	**44.5**	**16.1**	**68.4**	**38.9**	**60.2**
Local Range	**56.0 - 100.0**	**0.0 - 74.7**	**0.0- 66.9**	**12.4 - 100.0**	**0.0 - 90.9**	**35.1 - 86.2**

* Among schools that required health education.
† For example, science, social studies, home economics, or English.
‡ Survey did not include schools from the New York City Department of Education.
§ San Diego does not have a required health education course, but requires that health education be taught in science and physical education classes.

TABLE 3. Percentage of Schools That Taught a Required Health Education Course in Each Grade,* Selected U.S. Sites: School Health Profiles, Principal Surveys, 2006

Site	Grade 6	Grade 7	Grade 8	Grade 9	Grade 10	Grade 11	Grade 12
STATE SURVEYS							
Alabama	39.0	33.0	31.5	30.1	53.4	13.1	12.6
Alaska	39.0	42.8	44.0	65.9	44.5	42.3	34.9
Arizona	25.9	29.2	28.3	22.2	16.6	8.1	8.5
Arkansas	48.1	67.7	37.7	83.3	58.4	48.3	49.3
Connecticut	61.7	62.9	62.6	60.0	52.3	37.2	32.7
Delaware	61.4	79.8	73.6	63.0	32.2	14.6	11.7
Florida	29.9	28.9	29.9	39.0	25.9	19.0	17.2
Georgia	73.0	73.6	74.1	74.7	19.8	20.3	20.2
Hawaii	47.4	77.5	33.9	46.8	61.8	22.4	15.7
Idaho	35.9	62.0	63.0	16.9	56.1	35.5	11.2
Illinois	55.0	75.4	61.8	52.7	47.9	12.3	11.4
Iowa	33.3	40.9	40.2	35.5	30.3	16.6	14.4
Kansas	33.6	45.4	41.6	64.9	9.0	1.9	1.9
Maine	72.4	77.3	72.6	49.5	43.3	8.4	7.0
Massachusetts	58.2	65.0	66.9	52.1	40.2	19.9	15.2
Michigan	30.7	47.5	41.1	51.9	24.1	13.4	14.2
Mississippi	11.8	11.4	15.0	84.5	60.6	53.9	52.9
Missouri	52.0	68.4	67.3	67.9	16.6	11.1	11.0
Montana	71.1	85.9	88.1	86.1	82.4	8.6	7.3
Nebraska	44.4	58.5	58.8	55.8	30.3	8.5	7.2
New Hampshire	50.6	61.1	64.3	44.9	40.1	11.8	11.7
New York†	53.7	73.6	57.8	32.3	70.3	42.8	35.2
North Carolina	78.5	80.2	78.5	75.3	17.1	11.1	11.8
North Dakota	66.9	74.2	67.4	52.5	32.3	9.0	10.1
Oregon	77.0	81.7	83.4	67.0	64.8	40.6	21.3
Pennsylvania	71.2	72.8	73.0	54.3	51.1	53.5	23.4
Rhode Island	79.0	79.9	82.3	80.9	74.3	77.2	73.7
South Carolina	63.7	65.6	65.6	55.3	23.4	19.0	18.4
South Dakota	34.5	54.3	50.6	28.2	10.5	5.5	4.9
Tennessee	39.7	45.2	44.3	46.0	18.9	8.5	8.5
Texas	27.2	30.0	36.2	55.3	41.4	35.9	34.1
Utah	56.4	47.1	60.3	7.9	83.9	28.6	22.2
Vermont	48.5	55.7	51.9	44.0	24.1	15.3	14.9
Virginia	57.4	61.2	56.3	68.4	63.3	2.8	2.0
Washington	50.3	56.3	62.8	56.9	39.5	21.8	20.8
West Virginia	93.2	93.3	93.3	63.6	61.6	16.8	16.8
State Median	**51.3**	**62.5**	**61.1**	**54.8**	**40.8**	**16.7**	**14.7**
State Range	**11.8 - 93.2**	**11.4 - 93.3**	**15.0 - 93.3**	**7.9 - 86.1**	**9.0 - 83.9**	**1.9 - 77.2**	**1.9 - 73.7**

TABLE 3. Percentage of Schools That Taught a Required Health Education Course in Each Grade,* Selected U.S. Sites: School Health Profiles, Principal Surveys, 2006 *(continued)*

Site	Grade 6	Grade 7	Grade 8	Grade 9	Grade 10	Grade 11	Grade 12
LOCAL SURVEYS							
Charlotte-Mecklenburg County	100.0	100.0	100.0	100.0	39.7	11.1	11.1
Chicago	39.5	40.7	41.8	25.8	12.2	4.5	3.7
Dallas	4.2	18.5	14.8	31.6	42.8	35.6	33.3
District of Columbia	43.6	53.0	53.0	61.0	58.8	9.2	9.2
Hillsborough County	22.3	16.9	16.9	37.5	24.6	22.1	22.1
Los Angeles	48.5	93.5	4.6	97.3	10.0	6.9	6.9
Memphis	49.3	55.7	55.7	70.2	21.1	19.2	19.2
Miami	15.7	13.7	15.7	19.4	45.0	11.5	11.7
Orange County	0.0	4.8	0.0	35.3	11.2	8.4	8.4
Philadelphia	72.9	74.6	74.6	46.2	50.4	42.3	37.3
San Diego‡	0.0	0.0	0.0	0.0	0.0	0.0	0.0
San Francisco	34.6	33.2	33.2	29.3	18.5	13.3	9.3
Local Median	**37.1**	**37.0**	**25.1**	**36.4**	**22.9**	**11.3**	**10.2**
Local Range	**0.0 – 100.0**	**0.0 – 100.0**	**0.0 – 100.0**	**0.0 – 100.0**	**0.0 – 58.8**	**0.0 – 42.3**	**0.0 – 37.3**

* Among schools with students in that grade.
† Survey did not include schools from the New York City Department of Education.
‡ San Diego does not have a required health education course, but requires that health education be taught in science and physical education classes.

TABLE 4. Percentage of Schools That Required Teachers to Use Specific Materials in a Required Health Education Course, Selected U.S. Sites: School Health Profiles, Lead Health Education Teacher Surveys, 2006

Site	National Health Education Standards	State, district, or school developed curriculum	Commercially developed curriculum	Commercially developed student textbook	Commercially developed teacher's guide	Health education performance assessment materials	Materials from health organizations
STATE SURVEYS							
Alabama	39.7	75.4	33.3	54.7	45.2	37.5	45.6
Alaska	30.3	60.0	19.8	34.0	27.3	28.6	14.5
Arizona	24.7	36.3	15.0	20.7	21.4	23.1	20.5
Arkansas	65.6	91.6	38.6	76.5	62.4	54.1	41.8
Connecticut	60.8	75.1	18.4	18.9	19.2	47.0	29.6
Delaware	73.4	82.0	17.2	25.1	22.5	31.6	20.3
Florida	26.2	52.1	20.4	35.1	28.7	30.2	28.1
Georgia	39.9	86.8	42.7	67.6	62.8	46.0	41.8
Hawaii	64.4	56.4	18.0	20.2	15.8	46.1	21.5
Idaho	51.9	87.7	26.8	63.8	52.6	47.5	31.0
Iowa	33.6	61.0	20.1	35.9	30.2	25.5	27.0
Kansas	32.0	67.1	20.9	42.5	36.7	31.4	28.8
Maine	30.7	76.1	21.3	28.4	23.1	70.5	20.3
Massachusetts	46.2	71.8	33.7	24.4	29.3	39.1	36.2
Michigan	34.7	67.4	22.0	34.6	29.6	27.0	24.8
Mississippi	47.3	95.9	39.6	68.4	63.8	60.7	40.7
Missouri	44.8	80.3	20.9	53.3	43.6	54.6	34.2
Montana	57.6	86.5	26.6	43.4	38.4	42.6	38.2
Nebraska	35.8	65.4	27.3	50.9	42.4	28.9	33.6
New Hampshire	56.7	69.2	17.5	30.4	30.4	32.4	27.1
New York*	71.6	86.3	16.9	34.1	24.3	45.9	35.1
North Carolina	38.6	83.1	27.0	49.9	45.8	32.4	33.8
North Dakota	46.8	65.5	31.2	50.0	46.2	28.3	31.8
Oregon	57.4	76.9	36.0	46.9	39.7	30.5	24.6
Pennsylvania	63.0	84.6	19.2	50.9	37.4	38.5	37.5
Rhode Island	76.9	85.7	19.5	30.7	30.6	44.2	39.0
South Carolina	53.5	63.2	29.1	47.4	43.3	35.0	27.5
South Dakota	33.6	48.1	22.2	35.0	33.2	23.0	24.1
Tennessee	34.0	61.0	23.6	44.4	39.8	34.2	23.2
Texas	29.0	68.0	34.5	57.3	49.4	42.7	34.0
Utah	30.5	87.4	20.0	48.4	34.5	26.9	20.6
Vermont	43.3	49.5	27.4	17.6	25.0	24.4	17.6
Virginia	34.3	78.5	24.1	57.1	48.1	39.4	36.9
West Virginia	59.3	91.6	43.9	80.7	71.0	58.1	35.9
State Median	**44.1**	**75.3**	**22.9**	**43.9**	**37.1**	**36.3**	**30.3**
State Range	**24.7 - 76.9**	**36.3 - 95.9**	**15.0 - 43.9**	**17.6 - 80.7**	**15.8 - 71.0**	**23.0 - 70.5**	**14.5 - 45.6**

TABLE 4. Percentage of Schools That Required Teachers to Use Specific Materials in a Required Health Education Course, Selected U.S. Sites: School Health Profiles, Lead Health Education Teacher Surveys, 2006 *(continued)*

Site	National Health Education Standards	State, district, or school developed curriculum	Commercially developed curriculum	Commercially developed student textbook	Commercially developed teacher's guide	Health education performance assessment materials	Materials from health organizations
LOCAL SURVEYS							
Charlotte-Mecklenburg County	63.7	97.1	20.4	34.7	39.3	49.6	55.1
Chicago	29.8	39.4	20.8	28.6	31.6	23.6	24.0
Dallas	34.0	55.1	19.1	36.2	37.5	56.3	46.9
District of Columbia	49.1	47.2	25.2	53.9	51.8	55.8	31.2
Hillsborough County	16.6	39.3	12.3	30.6	26.5	20.0	21.7
Los Angeles	57.7	91.4	58.4	83.9	67.3	28.7	35.1
Memphis	62.8	77.8	40.4	71.1	62.6	59.2	30.1
Miami	32.5	47.5	14.1	30.4	22.8	22.9	36.8
Orange County	30.6	49.5	19.8	27.3	27.3	24.6	19.9
Philadelphia	58.3	77.5	29.3	43.5	39.5	46.6	42.7
San Diego†	0.0	0.0	0.0	0.0	0.0	0.0	0.0
San Francisco	25.9	48.2	35.7	28.6	32.1	17.9	17.9
Local Median	**33.3**	**48.9**	**20.6**	**32.7**	**34.8**	**26.7**	**30.7**
Local Range	**0.0 – 63.7**	**0.0 – 97.1**	**0.0 – 58.4**	**0.0 – 83.9**	**0.0 – 67.3**	**0.0 – 59.2**	**0.0 – 55.1**

* Survey did not include schools from the New York City Department of Education.

† San Diego does not have a required health education course, but requires that health education be taught in science and physical education classes.

TABLE 5a. Percentage of All Schools That Tried to Increase Student Knowledge on a Specific Health-Related Topic in a Required Health Education Course During the 2005–2006 School Year, Selected U.S. Sites: School Health Profiles, Lead Health Education Teacher Surveys, 2006

Site	Alcohol-use or other drug-use prevention	Asthma awareness	Consumer health	CPR*	Dental and oral health	Emotional and mental health	Environmental health
STATE SURVEYS							
Alabama	77.3	56.1	73.4	68.6	67.2	74.8	65.7
Alaska	73.8	35.3	61.9	42.7	58.9	67.2	51.4
Arizona	43.9	25.3	34.8	23.6	34.1	40.9	33.5
Arkansas	96.4	66.0	91.5	72.3	85.6	93.6	79.8
Connecticut	87.3	38.8	74.6	44.6	39.3	83.6	47.3
Delaware	90.5	51.8	77.1	46.8	49.1	85.3	52.8
Florida	55.9	28.3	48.2	41.8	37.1	52.3	37.7
Georgia	89.8	60.7	81.5	66.5	70.0	85.5	68.3
Hawaii	96.1	48.0	91.8	51.5	58.4	94.8	69.1
Idaho	94.9	61.3	88.4	69.0	70.5	92.9	72.0
Iowa	74.9	39.5	66.7	45.6	53.1	72.3	54.3
Kansas	75.9	36.1	64.1	44.3	50.0	68.9	50.8
Maine	90.3	39.1	83.7	53.4	48.3	85.4	60.8
Massachusetts	82.3	36.2	67.7	42.1	46.4	79.8	46.2
Michigan	76.3	35.4	65.2	33.2	42.9	73.0	43.2
Mississippi	97.9	64.1	95.5	78.6	87.4	96.0	80.8
Missouri	86.2	55.1	81.9	59.8	66.9	82.6	67.7
Montana	96.1	50.6	83.0	66.0	67.8	89.9	70.9
Nebraska	84.8	55.2	71.7	53.4	54.1	79.3	58.4
New Hampshire	85.4	38.1	78.9	44.1	53.9	81.4	60.1
New York†	99.0	61.3	93.8	66.2	64.6	98.4	74.3
North Carolina	87.3	63.1	77.7	65.0	54.5	84.4	67.4
North Dakota	89.5	54.4	81.2	62.5	69.8	84.3	66.6
Oregon	93.5	47.5	81.9	55.3	60.8	90.7	64.9
Pennsylvania	94.2	58.5	82.8	71.4	59.6	89.0	57.8
Rhode Island	96.5	48.5	86.8	49.5	46.0	92.9	60.0
South Carolina	70.0	41.6	57.9	40.1	50.1	65.4	50.7
South Dakota	68.2	35.4	58.8	47.1	49.5	60.6	44.2
Tennessee	70.3	46.1	58.9	49.2	51.9	66.0	50.7
Texas	78.6	49.9	70.7	65.5	59.9	75.5	63.7
Utah	94.8	45.0	80.1	62.1	55.9	92.6	59.8
Vermont	80.8	28.8	74.2	29.0	44.1	76.4	46.2
Virginia	83.5	51.7	73.3	58.5	59.7	81.0	57.6
West Virginia	98.3	71.6	90.9	67.1	81.4	96.7	83.2
State Median	**86.8**	**48.3**	**77.4**	**53.4**	**55.2**	**83.1**	**59.9**
State Range	**43.9 - 99.0**	**25.3 - 71.6**	**34.8 - 95.5**	**23.6 - 78.6**	**34.1 - 87.4**	**40.9 - 98.4**	**33.5 - 83.2**

TABLE 5a. Percentage of All Schools That Tried to Increase Student Knowledge on a Specific Health-Related Topic in a Required Health Education Course During the 2005–2006 School Year, Selected U.S. Sites: School Health Profiles, Lead Health Education Teacher Surveys, 2006 *(continued)*

Site	Alcohol-use or other drug-use prevention	Asthma awareness	Consumer health	CPR*	Dental and oral health	Emotional and mental health	Environmental health
LOCAL SURVEYS							
Charlotte-Mecklenburg County	100.0	67.2	91.9	68.3	40.3	97.4	62.1
Chicago	51.2	38.1	37.0	30.4	42.2	42.1	37.3
Dallas	58.0	29.2	56.0	58.0	42.9	57.1	57.1
District of Columbia	76.4	43.1	62.4	66.1	45.1	65.8	41.2
Hillsborough County	47.4	17.8	37.9	37.9	24.0	37.5	35.5
Los Angeles	100.0	76.8	95.0	57.6	91.7	98.9	84.8
Memphis	84.6	76.7	77.3	66.3	70.8	83.0	66.1
Miami	52.5	26.2	43.7	42.5	40.0	50.0	44.3
Orange County	49.5	22.2	41.2	40.6	24.9	49.5	35.9
Philadelphia	83.9	70.2	71.4	50.7	60.8	77.7	52.7
San Diego‡	0.0	0.0	0.0	0.0	0.0	0.0	0.0
San Francisco	57.2	35.7	48.2	25.0	33.3	57.2	50.0
Local Median	**57.6**	**36.9**	**52.1**	**46.6**	**41.3**	**57.2**	**47.2**
Local Range	**0.0 – 100.0**	**0.0 – 76.8**	**0.0 – 95.0**	**0.0 – 68.3**	**0.0 – 91.7**	**0.0 – 98.9**	**0.0 – 84.8**

* Cardiopulmonary resuscitation.
† Survey did not include schools from the New York City Department of Education.
‡ San Diego does not have a required health education course, but requires that health education be taught in science and physical education classes.

TABLE 5b. Percentage of All Schools That Tried to Increase Student Knowledge on a Specific Health-Related Topic in a Required Health Education Course During the 2005–2006 School Year, Selected U.S. Sites: School Health Profiles, Lead Health Education Teacher Surveys, 2006

Site	First aid	Foodborne illness prevention	Growth and development	HIV* prevention	Human sexuality	Immunizations	Injury prevention and safety
STATE SURVEYS							
Alabama	71.3	62.4	72.7	76.9	68.5	61.5	73.7
Alaska	51.9	51.4	66.4	69.3	61.9	51.7	63.6
Arizona	28.6	29.2	40.3	35.6	28.9	24.1	35.0
Arkansas	85.4	70.8	91.0	92.0	76.0	73.6	92.8
Connecticut	58.6	50.2	83.1	87.6	78.8	43.3	76.8
Delaware	68.8	60.2	84.4	88.1	83.8	42.6	83.5
Florida	39.4	42.6	53.6	55.2	52.1	33.3	46.2
Georgia	75.5	63.8	86.5	86.8	78.9	63.7	83.0
Hawaii	61.6	60.2	86.1	94.7	89.9	45.2	91.5
Idaho	81.6	76.6	85.9	92.8	77.5	69.2	86.6
Iowa	52.9	53.7	66.9	71.5	65.0	45.7	61.3
Kansas	49.5	53.0	71.2	74.7	70.3	39.3	63.1
Maine	61.0	57.4	83.4	86.6	79.2	45.9	78.4
Massachusetts	49.9	48.7	76.0	77.6	73.7	39.5	68.2
Michigan	44.9	46.9	70.1	76.4	67.4	33.5	62.2
Mississippi	88.2	84.5	94.1	97.9	84.8	79.4	90.1
Missouri	73.5	67.9	80.4	83.8	74.2	58.2	78.8
Montana	77.0	69.4	89.5	92.4	79.7	61.1	87.0
Nebraska	58.9	62.8	76.4	83.9	76.7	49.9	71.7
New Hampshire	55.0	61.3	80.8	84.3	78.5	52.8	73.3
New York†	77.1	74.1	96.5	99.3	96.9	73.9	88.8
North Carolina	71.9	64.5	75.3	84.0	70.5	46.4	82.2
North Dakota	73.6	71.4	82.4	84.4	73.9	66.9	79.1
Oregon	62.2	69.3	90.6	94.8	89.2	62.4	82.5
Pennsylvania	77.9	59.6	86.7	92.8	84.1	54.9	84.7
Rhode Island	60.5	61.7	89.1	96.3	89.2	55.4	84.5
South Carolina	53.0	51.0	64.9	69.5	65.7	45.1	63.5
South Dakota	52.1	43.5	55.2	61.0	51.1	36.6	57.5
Tennessee	59.0	52.2	62.6	65.7	62.0	47.4	65.0
Texas	68.9	64.2	75.3	73.6	64.5	54.2	73.1
Utah	70.0	62.6	88.1	92.2	84.0	53.7	84.0
Vermont	41.8	45.5	76.8	77.4	76.5	39.7	65.5
Virginia	69.5	61.4	78.2	78.1	72.7	50.2	74.0
West Virginia	81.5	83.3	90.8	94.7	86.0	76.8	93.9
State Median	**61.9**	**61.4**	**80.6**	**84.2**	**76.3**	**51.0**	**77.6**
State Range	**28.6 - 88.2**	**29.2 - 84.5**	**40.3 - 96.5**	**35.6 - 99.3**	**28.9 - 96.9**	**24.1 - 79.4**	**35.0 - 93.9**

TABLE 5b. Percentage of All Schools That Tried to Increase Student Knowledge on a Specific Health-Related Topic in a Required Health Education Course During the 2005–2006 School Year, Selected U.S. Sites: School Health Profiles, Lead Health Education Teacher Surveys, 2006 *(continued)*

Site	First aid	Foodborne illness prevention	Growth and development	HIV* prevention	Human sexuality	Immunizations	Injury prevention and safety
LOCAL SURVEYS							
Charlotte-Mecklenburg County	70.4	53.8	97.2	100.0	97.3	35.8	88.2
Chicago	38.0	33.2	48.6	45.2	42.3	33.9	45.7
Dallas	53.2	53.1	57.1	57.1	55.1	51.0	57.1
District of Columbia	58.5	48.8	68.5	75.5	66.1	54.4	65.8
Hillsborough County	34.1	35.6	40.8	45.7	42.2	25.7	37.6
Los Angeles	75.1	88.9	98.7	100.0	95.0	78.7	88.7
Memphis	80.8	65.4	83.0	84.6	82.8	62.9	84.6
Miami	42.5	41.7	51.2	52.5	48.7	38.7	47.5
Orange County	38.0	30.0	46.6	48.0	46.6	24.6	46.9
Philadelphia	70.9	50.0	80.8	81.3	76.5	51.0	74.3
San Diego‡	0.0	0.0	0.0	0.0	0.0	0.0	0.0
San Francisco	25.0	32.1	46.4	57.2	57.2	25.0	42.9
Local Median	**47.9**	**45.3**	**54.2**	**57.2**	**56.2**	**37.3**	**52.3**
Local Range	**0.0 – 80.8**	**0.0 – 88.9**	**0.0 – 98.7**	**0.0 – 100.0**	**0.0 – 97.3**	**0.0 – 78.7**	**0.0 – 88.7**

* Human immunodeficiency virus.
† Survey did not include schools from the New York City Department of Education.
‡ San Diego does not have a required health education course, but requires that health education be taught in science and physical education classes.

TABLE 5c. Percentage of All Schools That Tried to Increase Student Knowledge on a Specific Health-Related Topic in a Required Health Education Course During the 2005–2006 School Year, Selected U.S. Sites: School Health Profiles, Lead Health Education Teacher Surveys, 2006

Site	Nutrition and dietary behavior	Physical activity and fitness	Pregnancy prevention	STD* prevention	Suicide prevention	Sun safety or skin cancer prevention	Tobacco-use prevention	Violence prevention
STATE SURVEYS								
Alabama	76.6	77.1	75.1	74.6	69.3	66.2	77.3	74.8
Alaska	73.5	74.0	62.2	62.9	60.3	42.2	73.0	69.3
Arizona	43.1	44.0	29.6	30.8	32.6	37.3	42.9	39.7
Arkansas	95.9	96.0	87.1	86.4	78.8	78.9	95.5	91.3
Connecticut	85.4	86.4	84.3	83.2	69.3	56.9	87.1	80.8
Delaware	91.9	91.7	83.4	85.1	68.8	58.6	90.1	81.8
Florida	54.2	53.0	53.0	54.0	44.2	45.7	55.7	49.6
Georgia	88.7	89.2	83.8	84.3	66.4	73.6	89.8	79.5
Hawaii	96.1	96.1	92.0	92.3	72.9	64.9	96.1	91.1
Idaho	95.3	94.6	89.3	87.9	85.7	82.7	93.4	86.1
Iowa	73.4	73.5	68.6	69.8	58.4	63.0	74.2	61.7
Kansas	75.5	76.2	71.4	72.4	55.8	60.0	75.1	64.5
Maine	90.8	90.1	81.7	81.1	62.3	60.7	90.0	81.6
Massachusetts	81.4	81.1	74.1	74.1	61.0	66.0	81.2	77.9
Michigan	76.5	77.8	71.6	73.8	50.9	48.2	76.2	68.4
Mississippi	97.9	97.3	96.6	96.1	86.9	76.4	97.9	87.7
Missouri	86.1	85.7	80.0	81.1	65.6	73.3	85.9	75.1
Montana	95.4	95.5	87.4	83.2	72.4	69.7	95.5	88.7
Nebraska	85.4	86.7	78.2	77.0	62.9	65.0	86.2	65.8
New Hampshire	83.8	83.1	79.9	78.6	66.5	65.3	83.0	70.7
New York†	98.6	98.9	99.3	98.9	89.5	85.7	99.0	92.8
North Carolina	86.6	87.2	80.8	81.2	70.4	66.6	86.9	82.5
North Dakota	88.4	89.1	78.6	78.4	70.3	73.1	88.9	84.1
Oregon	93.2	94.2	93.2	90.2	75.3	69.5	94.9	85.6
Pennsylvania	92.8	94.1	89.8	89.3	64.4	70.2	93.8	80.7
Rhode Island	96.5	96.4	92.0	92.9	69.9	65.8	93.9	92.7
South Carolina	69.6	70.5	66.8	66.5	47.0	51.0	68.6	61.0
South Dakota	66.8	68.7	53.3	56.5	46.1	53.0	68.4	59.3
Tennessee	68.9	70.5	63.3	62.5	53.1	51.6	69.6	63.4
Texas	78.3	78.7	70.5	70.2	64.9	66.3	78.6	70.9
Utah	94.7	94.7	85.3	85.7	88.3	69.2	94.8	86.3
Vermont	79.4	76.6	75.2	75.2	53.9	49.4	80.8	73.7
Virginia	83.2	83.4	74.1	74.8	59.6	66.9	82.2	77.1
West Virginia	97.7	97.7	92.6	93.2	80.5	84.2	98.3	95.3
State Median	**85.8**	**86.5**	**80.0**	**79.9**	**66.0**	**65.9**	**86.6**	**78.7**
State Range	**43.1 - 98.6**	**44.0 - 98.9**	**29.6 - 99.3**	**30.8 - 98.9**	**32.6 - 89.5**	**37.3 - 85.7**	**42.9 - 99.0**	**39.7 - 95.3**

TABLE 5c. Percentage of All Schools That Tried to Increase Student Knowledge on a Specific Health-Related Topic in a Required Health Education Course During the 2005–2006 School Year, Selected U.S. Sites: School Health Profiles, Lead Health Education Teacher Surveys, 2006 *(continued)*

Site	Nutrition and dietary behavior	Physical activity and fitness	Pregnancy prevention	STD* prevention	Suicide prevention	Sun safety or skin cancer prevention	Tobacco-use prevention	Violence prevention
LOCAL SURVEYS								
Charlotte-Mecklenburg County	97.3	100.0	100.0	100.0	91.9	69.7	97.3	94.4
Chicago	50.9	52.2	39.8	41.4	29.4	29.2	48.3	45.4
Dallas	57.1	55.3	55.1	57.1	55.1	46.9	57.1	57.1
District of Columbia	71.7	75.5	69.7	68.5	48.5	32.4	71.0	62.4
Hillsborough County	42.8	42.0	39.2	44.0	36.7	41.4	45.8	42.8
Los Angeles	100.0	100.0	100.0	96.2	81.1	87.9	100.0	95.2
Memphis	82.2	84.6	84.4	82.4	67.5	53.8	83.8	82.4
Miami	50.6	50.6	52.5	52.5	46.3	42.6	51.9	46.2
Orange County	46.6	46.4	46.6	46.6	40.6	43.9	49.5	44.2
Philadelphia	84.4	82.8	75.4	76.2	50.6	46.3	82.5	76.9
San Diego‡	0.0	0.0	0.0	0.0	0.0	0.0	0.0	0.0
San Francisco	57.2	57.2	57.2	57.2	50.0	32.2	57.2	57.2
Local Median	**57.2**	**56.3**	**56.2**	**57.2**	**49.3**	**43.3**	**57.2**	**57.2**
Local Range	**0.0 – 100.0**	**0.0 – 100.0**	**0.0 – 100.0**	**0.0 – 100.0**	**0.0 – 91.9**	**0.0 – 87.9**	**0.0 – 100.0**	**0.0 – 95.2**

* Sexually transmitted disease.
† Survey did not include schools from the New York City Department of Education.
‡ San Diego does not have a required health education course, but requires that health education be taught in science and physical education classes.

TABLE 6. Percentage of All Schools That Tried To Improve Specific Student Skills in a Required Health Education Course During the 2005–2006 School Year, Selected U.S. Sites: School Health Profiles, Lead Health Education Teacher Surveys, 2006

Site	Finding valid information or services related to personal health and wellness	Influence of media on personal health and wellness	Communication skills	Decision-making skills	Goal-setting skills	Conflict resolution skills	Resisting peer pressure to engage in unhealthy behaviors
STATE SURVEYS							
Alabama	72.9	69.7	71.9	74.8	75.1	74.3	77.0
Alaska	63.6	58.8	58.3	56.7	67.3	66.5	70.7
Arizona	35.7	37.6	36.8	34.6	40.3	39.1	42.0
Arkansas	89.2	91.4	87.2	87.9	94.2	88.5	96.0
Connecticut	79.7	83.3	80.7	79.3	80.4	81.2	87.7
Delaware	83.8	86.9	83.2	88.3	88.3	86.6	91.7
Florida	49.7	52.0	51.5	51.3	52.8	52.9	55.1
Georgia	83.7	83.4	81.1	81.3	88.7	81.8	89.4
Hawaii	90.0	93.1	91.3	89.4	96.1	88.2	96.1
Idaho	85.4	89.0	86.6	87.2	92.0	89.1	92.5
Iowa	65.0	67.3	62.5	63.2	69.2	63.3	71.9
Kansas	65.4	67.0	59.4	63.8	70.7	65.1	75.2
Maine	83.2	86.7	82.5	79.8	87.0	81.2	89.3
Massachusetts	75.8	78.4	75.6	75.7	78.2	75.6	81.6
Michigan	67.3	72.3	64.7	65.7	70.8	69.3	75.3
Mississippi	95.3	87.4	93.7	91.0	92.7	91.1	97.3
Missouri	79.8	80.4	75.5	77.6	83.0	78.1	85.2
Montana	81.4	86.9	82.0	79.8	92.4	87.4	95.0
Nebraska	75.7	78.6	67.1	76.7	81.4	68.4	86.2
New Hampshire	79.5	80.8	80.8	76.5	79.0	70.9	84.1
New York*	96.7	96.7	94.1	94.9	98.0	90.3	98.8
North Carolina	78.1	79.5	77.2	78.1	84.4	83.3	85.8
North Dakota	78.8	80.7	77.2	80.5	81.5	81.5	86.2
Oregon	85.5	90.9	80.6	82.9	90.4	88.0	93.3
Pennsylvania	85.8	87.4	83.4	83.3	88.5	84.8	93.0
Rhode Island	89.3	94.1	92.9	92.9	95.3	94.0	94.1
South Carolina	62.8	61.7	65.2	63.5	68.0	63.6	68.3
South Dakota	54.7	56.7	48.7	47.1	60.5	55.3	66.5
Tennessee	60.5	59.6	61.7	60.8	65.6	65.3	68.5
Texas	70.8	69.6	69.7	70.6	77.0	71.0	76.8
Utah	81.2	93.3	84.5	87.1	93.5	87.4	94.3
Vermont	71.8	78.1	75.3	71.0	77.4	70.1	78.0
Virginia	73.1	75.2	71.5	70.5	80.5	76.1	82.1
West Virginia	94.6	96.5	92.4	94.9	96.1	95.6	97.9
State Median	**79.2**	**80.6**	**77.2**	**77.9**	**81.5**	**79.7**	**86.0**
State Range	**35.7 - 96.7**	**37.6 - 96.7**	**36.8 - 94.1**	**34.6 - 94.9**	**40.3 - 98.0**	**39.1 - 95.6**	**42.0 - 98.8**

TABLE 6. Percentage of All Schools That Tried To Improve Specific Student Skills in a Required Health Education Course During the 2005–2006 School Year, Selected U.S. Sites: School Health Profiles, Lead Health Education Teacher Surveys, 2006 *(continued)*

Site	Finding valid information or services related to personal health and wellness	Influence of media on personal health and wellness	Communication skills	Decision-making skills	Goal-setting skills	Conflict resolution skills	Resisting peer pressure to engage in unhealthy behaviors
LOCAL SURVEYS							
Charlotte-Mecklenburg County	97.2	94.5	100.0	92.1	97.4	94.5	100.0
Chicago	43.0	38.0	43.7	40.5	46.6	47.4	48.3
Dallas	55.1	55.1	55.1	57.1	55.1	57.1	57.1
District of Columbia	76.4	58.8	69.4	69.7	76.4	69.1	72.7
Hillsborough County	37.5	39.6	37.5	37.5	44.7	46.5	44.7
Los Angeles	91.4	97.5	90.3	91.2	90.4	92.9	98.9
Memphis	78.7	83.0	81.9	79.0	80.4	82.7	84.4
Miami	48.8	47.5	50.0	51.3	50.0	48.7	51.2
Orange County	49.5	49.5	46.6	49.5	49.5	46.9	49.5
Philadelphia	67.5	73.3	68.7	69.8	76.7	77.1	83.0
San Diego†	0.0	0.0	0.0	0.0	0.0	0.0	0.0
San Francisco	53.6	53.6	53.6	57.2	53.6	57.2	53.6
Local Median	**54.4**	**54.4**	**54.4**	**57.2**	**54.4**	**57.2**	**55.4**
Local Range	**0.0 – 97.2**	**0.0 – 97.5**	**0.0 – 100.0**	**0.0 – 92.1**	**0.0 – 97.4**	**0.0 – 94.5**	**0.0 – 100.0**

* Survey did not include schools from the New York City Department of Education.
† San Diego does not have a required health education course, but requires that health education be taught in science and physical education classes.

TABLE 7a. Percentage of All Schools That Taught About Health Outcomes and Risks of Tobacco Use in a Required Health Education Course During the 2005–2006 School Year, Selected U.S. Sites: School Health Profiles, Lead Health Education Teacher Surveys, 2006

Site	Addictive effects of nicotine	Benefits of not smoking cigarettes	Benefits of not using smokeless tobacco	Short-term and long-term health consequences of cigarette smoking	Short-term and long-term health consequences of using smokeless tobacco	Health effects of ETS* or second-hand smoke	Short-term and long-term health consequences of cigar smoking
STATE SURVEYS							
Alabama	76.6	76.6	73.5	77.1	74.3	75.0	72.5
Alaska	70.7	71.7	68.3	71.4	67.9	66.3	50.7
Arizona	40.8	42.0	37.6	41.3	38.5	40.2	35.9
Arkansas	94.7	95.6	94.8	95.6	95.1	93.3	88.5
Connecticut	86.3	86.0	81.3	86.7	83.8	85.6	68.8
Delaware	90.1	88.5	86.9	88.7	87.1	87.0	80.0
Florida	53.6	54.7	50.4	54.7	50.9	53.5	47.3
Georgia	89.7	89.7	88.5	89.7	88.6	89.3	83.4
Hawaii	92.5	96.1	84.6	96.1	88.8	89.9	76.2
Idaho	93.4	94.0	92.3	94.0	92.8	93.3	85.6
Iowa	71.6	73.4	68.4	73.8	68.6	70.7	57.7
Kansas	71.8	73.5	72.7	73.6	74.0	71.7	63.0
Maine	88.5	88.5	81.5	88.5	82.7	86.6	65.3
Massachusetts	79.6	79.0	73.8	79.5	75.4	78.5	65.6
Michigan	73.7	74.6	72.3	75.0	73.0	73.7	65.7
Mississippi	96.7	97.9	96.8	97.3	96.8	96.0	90.5
Missouri	83.3	85.0	80.6	85.0	81.0	82.8	72.0
Montana	93.8	94.5	92.4	93.8	93.8	93.0	79.0
Nebraska	84.9	85.7	81.9	85.7	84.4	82.3	68.3
New Hampshire	80.8	81.9	79.6	82.5	79.5	80.0	72.4
New York†	99.0	98.7	95.9	99.0	98.1	97.9	91.0
North Carolina	86.7	86.3	84.3	86.7	84.9	85.6	77.4
North Dakota	87.6	87.6	85.6	87.6	86.3	87.4	75.3
Oregon	93.2	93.4	87.3	93.5	91.0	92.1	71.3
Pennsylvania	91.9	92.7	89.9	92.8	91.3	91.7	82.0
Rhode Island	92.8	92.8	88.2	94.0	89.4	90.5	74.4
South Carolina	66.5	66.9	64.4	66.5	65.2	66.5	58.1
South Dakota	65.4	66.4	64.2	66.9	65.5	64.5	52.4
Tennessee	67.1	69.1	65.9	68.6	67.7	66.8	61.9
Texas	76.8	77.5	76.9	77.5	77.2	76.0	71.4
Utah	92.3	94.2	89.7	94.7	90.7	92.4	75.6
Vermont	78.1	78.1	75.2	79.1	76.4	75.5	64.0
Virginia	80.3	81.5	77.9	81.5	78.0	79.4	67.9
West Virginia	97.7	98.3	98.3	98.3	98.3	98.3	90.3
State Median	**85.6**	**85.9**	**81.4**	**86.2**	**83.3**	**84.2**	**71.7**
State Range	**40.8 - 99.0**	**42.0 - 98.7**	**37.6 - 98.3**	**41.3 - 99.0**	**38.5 - 98.3**	**40.2 - 98.3**	**35.9 - 91.0**

TABLE 7a. Percentage of All Schools That Taught About Health Outcomes and Risks of Tobacco Use in a Required Health Education Course During the 2005–2006 School Year, Selected U.S. Sites: School Health Profiles, Lead Health Education Teacher Surveys, 2006 *(continued)*

Site	Addictive effects of nicotine	Benefits of not smoking cigarettes	Benefits of not using smokeless tobacco	Short-term and long-term health consequences of cigarette smoking	Short-term and long-term health consequences of using smokeless tobacco	Health effects of ETS* or second-hand smoke	Short-term and long-term health consequences of cigar smoking
LOCAL SURVEYS							
Charlotte-Mecklenburg County	97.4	97.4	89.3	97.4	91.9	94.7	81.0
Chicago	45.2	47.6	33.8	47.6	34.9	47.1	36.5
Dallas	56.3	56.3	56.3	56.3	54.2	55.3	52.1
District of Columbia	68.5	68.5	48.5	68.5	55.8	64.8	52.4
Hillsborough County	43.1	44.0	43.1	44.0	43.1	43.1	39.0
Los Angeles	100.0	100.0	98.7	100.0	97.5	98.9	93.9
Memphis	80.3	81.9	73.8	79.5	73.8	77.3	70.0
Miami	48.1	50.0	44.3	50.0	44.3	49.4	45.6
Orange County	46.6	46.6	46.6	46.6	46.6	46.6	41.2
Philadelphia	77.8	79.6	64.2	80.9	69.2	77.6	67.0
San Diego‡	0.0	0.0	0.0	0.0	0.0	0.0	0.0
San Francisco	57.2	57.2	50.0	57.2	53.6	53.6	32.1
Local Median	**56.8**	**56.8**	**49.3**	**56.8**	**53.9**	**54.5**	**48.9**
Local Range	**0.0 – 100.0**	**0.0 – 100.0**	**0.0 – 98.7**	**0.0 – 100.0**	**0.0 – 97.5**	**0.0 – 98.9**	**0.0 – 93.9**

* Environmental tobacco smoke.
† Survey did not include schools from the New York City Department of Education.
‡ San Diego does not have a required health education course, but requires that health education be taught in science and physical education classes.

TABLE 7b. Percentage of All Schools That Taught About External Influences on Tobacco Use in a Required Health Education Course During the 2005–2006 School Year, Selected U.S. Sites: School Health Profiles, Lead Health Education Teacher Surveys, 2006

Site	Influence of families on tobacco use	Influence of the media on tobacco use	Social or cultural influences on tobacco use	How many young people use tobacco
STATE SURVEYS				
Alabama	74.3	74.4	73.6	73.8
Alaska	64.8	66.1	63.5	67.8
Arizona	35.7	38.1	36.5	37.2
Arkansas	93.4	93.0	91.4	93.8
Connecticut	82.2	84.2	78.2	80.6
Delaware	90.1	90.1	83.5	85.1
Florida	51.2	53.9	51.0	51.7
Georgia	88.2	89.0	85.1	88.0
Hawaii	88.8	94.8	89.1	91.7
Idaho	91.2	91.2	88.6	90.8
Iowa	67.2	69.0	65.7	68.0
Kansas	70.3	70.9	66.8	69.5
Maine	83.7	85.5	76.4	79.6
Massachusetts	74.6	78.7	72.8	75.3
Michigan	71.2	73.7	69.0	70.1
Mississippi	95.2	94.0	91.5	94.1
Missouri	79.2	81.3	79.8	78.7
Montana	91.3	91.7	91.0	89.7
Nebraska	82.2	83.5	79.3	81.8
New Hampshire	78.2	80.5	73.6	76.8
New York*	96.4	98.7	94.9	96.2
North Carolina	82.9	86.4	81.9	83.9
North Dakota	82.6	85.2	80.2	83.3
Oregon	89.2	92.7	86.3	87.0
Pennsylvania	89.4	91.7	85.1	90.2
Rhode Island	86.9	89.4	87.0	89.2
South Carolina	63.6	63.7	62.5	64.1
South Dakota	63.7	65.2	60.4	62.2
Tennessee	63.3	64.3	63.1	63.8
Texas	72.8	76.0	71.3	73.7
Utah	89.1	93.6	85.1	86.1
Vermont	69.6	75.4	72.0	70.0
Virginia	77.9	78.5	74.4	76.4
West Virginia	97.1	97.7	95.0	96.6
State Median	**82.2**	**83.9**	**78.8**	**80.1**
State Range	**35.7 - 97.1**	**38.1 - 98.7**	**36.5 - 95.0**	**37.2 - 96.6**

TABLE 7b. Percentage of All Schools That Taught About External Influences on Tobacco Use in a Required Health Education Course During the 2005–2006 School Year, Selected U.S. Sites: School Health Profiles, Lead Health Education Teacher Surveys, 2006 *(continued)*

Site	Influence of families on tobacco use	Influence of the media on tobacco use	Social or cultural influences on tobacco use	How many young people use tobacco
LOCAL SURVEYS				
Charlotte-Mecklenburg County	94.5	91.7	89.1	94.7
Chicago	40.4	41.0	39.2	40.7
Dallas	56.3	56.3	56.3	54.2
District of Columbia	67.1	67.1	59.1	67.1
Hillsborough County	43.1	43.1	41.0	43.1
Los Angeles	97.6	100.0	96.3	96.6
Memphis	80.1	77.8	78.4	74.9
Miami	48.1	49.4	48.2	48.1
Orange County	43.9	46.6	43.9	46.6
Philadelphia	76.0	77.8	73.4	74.9
San Diego†	0.0	0.0	0.0	0.0
San Francisco	50.0	57.2	57.2	57.2
Local Median	**53.2**	**56.8**	**56.8**	**55.7**
Local Range	**0.0 – 97.6**	**0.0 – 100.0**	**0.0 – 96.3**	**0.0 – 96.6**

* Survey did not include schools from the New York City Department of Education.

† San Diego does not have a required health education course, but requires that health education be taught in science and physical education classes.

TABLE 7c. Percentage of All Schools That Taught Skills to Avoid and to Stop Using Tobacco in a Required Health Education Course During the 2005–2006 School Year, Selected U.S. Sites: School Health Profiles, Lead Health Education Teacher Surveys, 2006

Site	Resisting peer pressure to use tobacco	Making a personal commitment not to use tobacco	How students can influence or support others to prevent tobacco use	How to find valid information or services related to tobacco-use prevention or cessation	How students can influence or support others in efforts to quit using tobacco
STATE SURVEYS					
Alabama	76.8	64.3	75.2	70.4	74.0
Alaska	69.0	51.1	61.8	57.3	62.1
Arizona	40.0	32.2	36.7	33.1	35.5
Arkansas	95.6	75.5	90.8	80.8	90.5
Connecticut	83.9	57.9	77.1	68.2	74.2
Delaware	90.1	64.6	79.8	81.7	76.3
Florida	54.0	42.7	50.3	48.2	50.5
Georgia	88.9	75.0	87.4	79.1	88.1
Hawaii	96.1	68.5	88.4	77.8	88.4
Idaho	92.8	73.9	86.9	80.5	89.0
Iowa	69.6	51.7	65.9	59.4	63.7
Kansas	73.1	47.1	65.9	55.5	64.4
Maine	87.6	57.4	77.3	67.5	78.2
Massachusetts	78.5	60.1	72.1	64.6	70.1
Michigan	73.9	50.1	68.9	58.4	67.5
Mississippi	96.7	80.6	93.5	89.3	92.7
Missouri	83.1	64.3	79.2	70.3	78.4
Montana	93.2	75.8	87.0	77.7	86.8
Nebraska	83.5	63.0	78.2	64.5	74.3
New Hampshire	77.4	60.1	70.3	67.1	68.9
New York*	97.5	79.7	93.6	89.0	93.4
North Carolina	85.6	70.8	81.3	72.8	79.8
North Dakota	86.8	68.4	84.8	72.3	78.5
Oregon	92.2	66.0	87.0	71.7	84.6
Pennsylvania	92.9	71.7	84.9	77.2	83.0
Rhode Island	89.4	75.7	86.9	79.4	83.4
South Carolina	68.6	55.3	64.0	56.7	63.1
South Dakota	65.6	47.9	59.9	51.3	61.0
Tennessee	67.2	53.4	59.7	53.0	61.5
Texas	77.2	58.6	73.8	66.1	72.6
Utah	93.7	77.2	89.7	74.4	88.6
Vermont	76.7	48.7	66.9	62.9	62.2
Virginia	80.5	63.9	74.1	66.7	74.1
West Virginia	97.9	84.5	96.8	93.2	95.1
State Median	**83.7**	**64.1**	**77.8**	**69.3**	**75.3**
State Range	**40.0 - 97.9**	**32.2 - 84.5**	**36.7 - 96.8**	**33.1 - 93.2**	**35.5 - 95.1**

TABLE 7c. Percentage of All Schools That Taught Skills to Avoid and to Stop Using Tobacco in a Required Health Education Course During the 2005–2006 School Year, Selected U.S. Sites: School Health Profiles, Lead Health Education Teacher Surveys, 2006 *(continued)*

Site	Resisting peer pressure to use tobacco	Making a personal commitment not to use tobacco	How students can influence or support others to prevent tobacco use	How to find valid information or services related to tobacco-use prevention or cessation	How students can influence or support others in efforts to quit using tobacco
LOCAL SURVEYS					
Charlotte-Mecklenburg County	97.4	67.4	89.3	75.9	86.6
Chicago	45.2	36.2	41.6	33.2	39.3
Dallas	56.3	47.9	52.1	47.9	52.1
District of Columbia	68.5	57.7	67.1	51.8	71.0
Hillsborough County	43.1	37.0	39.0	43.1	41.0
Los Angeles	98.9	86.9	97.7	92.7	95.3
Memphis	77.6	70.2	77.9	58.6	78.4
Miami	49.4	43.0	49.4	48.1	50.7
Orange County	46.6	38.6	41.2	39.6	46.6
Philadelphia	79.8	59.8	68.1	62.4	69.0
San Diego†	0.0	0.0	0.0	0.0	0.0
San Francisco	57.2	50.0	57.2	53.6	57.2
Local Median	**56.8**	**49.0**	**54.7**	**50.0**	**54.7**
Local Range	**0.0 - 98.9**	**0.0 - 86.9**	**0.0 - 97.7**	**0.0 - 92.7**	**0.0 - 95.3**

* Survey did not include schools from the New York City Department of Education.

† San Diego does not have a required health education course, but requires that health education be taught in science and physical education classes.

TABLE 8a. Percentage of All Schools That Taught About HIV* Transmission and Prevention in a Required Health Education Course During the 2005–2006 School Year, Selected U.S. Sites: School Health Profiles, Lead Health Education Teacher Surveys, 2006

Site	Abstinence as the most effective method to avoid pregnancy, HIV, and STDs†	How HIV is transmitted	How HIV affects the human body	Condom efficacy	Risks associated with having multiple sexual partners
STATE SURVEYS					
Alabama	74.0	74.7	74.4	60.3	70.9
Alaska	58.3	60.4	58.6	44.0	56.2
Arizona	28.5	28.0	28.3	20.0	26.5
Arkansas	85.9	84.9	83.1	56.3	79.7
Connecticut	82.3	84.1	82.8	68.5	75.1
Delaware	87.9	83.1	83.1	71.2	83.2
Florida	52.0	51.8	51.3	40.9	50.2
Georgia	84.0	84.5	83.3	62.6	80.1
Hawaii	93.1	91.8	89.9	76.2	88.0
Idaho	88.9	87.6	85.1	51.6	78.8
Iowa	67.4	67.9	67.5	55.6	65.7
Kansas	69.1	69.7	67.7	49.1	64.7
Maine	80.9	81.2	79.7	65.5	74.5
Massachusetts	72.0	73.1	72.0	58.7	66.8
Michigan	69.8	70.5	70.1	49.3	64.8
Mississippi	97.0	97.2	95.8	74.2	93.8
Missouri	78.7	80.2	79.9	51.1	71.9
Montana	84.9	84.0	83.0	59.3	78.3
Nebraska	76.8	77.1	73.8	54.1	70.3
New Hampshire	77.3	79.0	78.3	61.9	74.4
New York‡	99.3	99.3	99.3	90.0	96.2
North Carolina	81.0	78.4	76.4	50.5	67.6
North Dakota	76.9	77.8	77.2	47.2	74.1
Oregon	91.5	91.6	91.4	76.7	83.6
Pennsylvania	88.4	89.0	89.0	67.0	84.7
Rhode Island	92.0	93.4	93.4	68.2	85.8
South Carolina	65.9	65.8	64.9	45.6	59.4
South Dakota	50.3	50.1	48.9	28.4	43.3
Tennessee	61.5	62.4	61.2	47.2	59.7
Texas	69.2	67.4	66.8	44.0	62.6
Utah	87.5	87.0	85.5	31.5	75.4
Vermont	72.2	74.0	71.5	65.4	73.2
Virginia	72.4	73.1	72.9	11.7	66.0
West Virginia	92.4	91.1	91.1	72.6	86.8
State Median	**78.0**	**78.7**	**77.8**	**56.0**	**73.7**
State Range	**28.5 - 99.3**	**28.0 - 99.3**	**28.3 - 99.3**	**11.7 - 90.0**	**26.5 - 96.2**

TABLE 8a. Percentage of All Schools That Taught About HIV* Transmission and Prevention in a Required Health Education Course During the 2005–2006 School Year, Selected U.S. Sites: School Health Profiles, Lead Health Education Teacher Surveys, 2006 *(continued)*

Site	Abstinence as the most effective method to avoid pregnancy, HIV, and STDs†	How HIV is transmitted	How HIV affects the human body	Condom efficacy	Risks associated with having multiple sexual partners
LOCAL SURVEYS					
Charlotte-Mecklenburg County	100.0	100.0	97.3	83.4	91.7
Chicago	37.4	39.4	39.5	31.0	35.6
Dallas	56.3	54.2	54.2	35.4	54.2
District of Columbia	71.0	71.0	71.0	60.2	71.0
Hillsborough County	39.2	39.2	39.2	34.0	38.5
Los Angeles	97.4	98.7	98.7	91.1	95.0
Memphis	84.4	84.4	84.4	65.6	84.4
Miami	52.5	52.5	51.2	50.0	52.5
Orange County	48.0	46.6	46.6	43.6	46.6
Philadelphia	75.4	74.1	72.0	56.0	73.4
San Diego§	0.0	0.0	0.0	0.0	0.0
San Francisco	57.2	57.2	57.2	57.2	57.2
Local Median	**56.8**	**55.7**	**55.7**	**53.0**	**55.7**
Local Range	**0.0 - 100.0**	**0.0 - 100.0**	**0.0 - 98.7**	**0.0 - 91.1**	**0.0 - 95.0**

* Human immunodeficiency virus.
† Sexually transmitted disease.
‡ Survey did not include schools from the New York City Department of Education.
§ San Diego does not have a required health education course, but requires that health education be taught in science and physical education classes.

TABLE 8b. Percentage of All Schools That Taught About External Influences on Behaviors Related to HIV* Infection, and Skills to Avoid HIV Infection, STDs,† and Pregnancy in a Required Health Education Course During the 2005–2006 School Year, Selected U.S. Sites: School Health Profiles, Lead Health Education Teacher Surveys, 2006

Site	Influence of alcohol and other drugs on HIV-related risk behaviors	Social or cultural influences on sexual behavior	How to prevent HIV infection	How to find valid information or services related to HIV or HIV testing	How to correctly use a condom	Compassion for persons living with HIV or AIDS‡
STATE SURVEYS						
Alabama	73.5	67.3	74.2	68.0	21.5	65.3
Alaska	55.7	52.7	60.0	49.6	22.3	44.3
Arizona	26.8	24.1	27.6	22.9	9.6	23.3
Arkansas	83.3	71.3	83.4	72.8	19.5	71.4
Connecticut	82.6	65.6	83.8	62.9	39.7	73.9
Delaware	82.8	74.4	83.1	76.3	43.8	71.6
Florida	50.8	46.0	51.9	46.3	25.5	45.2
Georgia	81.6	72.5	84.0	74.8	19.0	73.2
Hawaii	89.3	82.2	91.8	82.8	51.6	84.4
Idaho	85.9	65.4	87.6	69.3	18.4	69.2
Iowa	63.8	59.3	67.4	52.8	28.6	54.7
Kansas	66.9	55.1	69.0	51.8	20.4	54.2
Maine	77.6	63.5	80.1	68.8	45.4	65.2
Massachusetts	70.7	61.0	72.5	60.8	36.4	65.3
Michigan	67.7	57.2	70.4	55.9	23.1	60.4
Mississippi	95.1	86.9	97.2	87.8	28.9	84.4
Missouri	77.4	65.3	79.9	65.2	19.0	64.6
Montana	87.3	67.7	84.4	75.3	29.2	71.2
Nebraska	76.5	62.6	75.8	55.4	19.4	59.6
New Hampshire	79.1	68.4	78.4	67.7	42.5	71.0
New York§	99.3	87.7	98.9	91.9	59.1	91.6
North Carolina	76.4	62.9	78.0	60.0	12.8	63.7
North Dakota	76.2	67.6	77.8	65.5	15.8	68.7
Oregon	88.8	79.5	91.6	70.4	44.5	75.0
Pennsylvania	87.1	70.1	88.7	72.8	36.2	75.9
Rhode Island	90.8	75.7	89.7	82.2	43.6	82.0
South Carolina	62.5	55.8	65.0	56.8	26.3	55.9
South Dakota	48.3	42.7	50.4	35.7	11.6	32.9
Tennessee	59.0	55.7	62.0	55.2	17.7	51.8
Texas	64.5	57.0	66.5	56.1	16.5	55.1
Utah	80.2	69.3	85.7	56.4	1.0	74.1
Vermont	70.1	60.2	74.0	60.8	46.0	65.7
Virginia	71.5	56.1	72.5	62.8	7.7	61.1
West Virginia	89.2	82.9	92.4	81.3	33.6	81.5
State Median	**77.0**	**65.4**	**78.2**	**64.1**	**24.3**	**65.5**
State Range	**26.8 – 99.3**	**24.1 – 87.7**	**27.6 – 98.9**	**22.9 – 91.9**	**1.0 – 59.1**	**23.3 – 91.6**

TABLE 8b. Percentage of All Schools That Taught About External Influences on Behaviors Related to HIV* Infection, and Skills to Avoid HIV Infection, STDs,† and Pregnancy in a Required Health Education Course During the 2005–2006 School Year, Selected U.S. Sites: School Health Profiles, Lead Health Education Teacher Surveys, 2006 *(continued)*

Site	Influence of alcohol and other drugs on HIV-related risk behaviors	Social or cultural influences on sexual behavior	How to prevent HIV infection	How to find valid information or services related to HIV or HIV testing	How to correctly use a condom	Compassion for persons living with HIV or AIDS‡
LOCAL SURVEYS						
Charlotte-Mecklenburg County	97.3	86.1	97.3	72.8	22.0	75.1
Chicago	37.1	32.4	39.0	33.6	18.5	37.1
Dallas	52.1	50.0	54.2	52.1	12.5	50.0
District of Columbia	71.0	64.8	71.0	67.1	44.0	64.8
Hillsborough County	39.2	37.6	39.2	38.4	18.2	36.2
Los Angeles	97.4	90.1	98.7	92.3	74.8	88.8
Memphis	84.4	83.0	84.4	81.9	33.7	80.1
Miami	51.3	48.7	52.5	51.2	42.4	51.2
Orange County	43.9	40.9	46.6	46.6	34.7	43.9
Philadelphia	68.1	60.6	73.2	61.0	37.5	63.9
San Diego‖	0.0	0.0	0.0	0.0	0.0	0.0
San Francisco	57.2	46.4	57.2	53.6	42.9	53.6
Local Median	**54.7**	**49.4**	**55.7**	**52.9**	**34.2**	**52.4**
Local Range	**0.0 - 97.4**	**0.0 - 90.1**	**0.0 - 98.7**	**0.0 - 92.3**	**0.0 - 74.8**	**0.0 - 88.8**

* Human immunodeficiency virus.
† Sexually transmitted disease.
‡ Acquired immunodeficiency syndrome.
§ Survey did not include schools from the New York City Department of Education.
‖ San Diego does not have a required health education course, but requires that health education be taught in science and physical education classes.

TABLE 9. Percentage of All Schools That Taught Required HIV* Prevention Units or Lessons in Specific Courses, Selected U.S. Sites: School Health Profiles, Lead Health Education Teacher Surveys, 2006

Site	Science	Home economics or family and consumer education	Physical education	Family life education or life skills	Special education	Social studies
STATE SURVEYS						
Alabama	66.3	45.3	53.2	45.1	30.6	18.3
Alaska	29.1	11.0	22.6	31.7	9.8	12.1
Arizona	26.0	7.2	19.7	16.9	7.9	7.2
Arkansas	44.1	53.4	31.5	55.9	28.2	12.5
Connecticut	32.5	12.4	20.3	41.4	15.0	6.8
Delaware	22.8	15.9	22.4	29.1	20.0	5.4
Florida	54.2	28.1	27.7	52.0	26.1	12.4
Georgia	35.2	25.5	45.8	36.5	24.4	7.7
Hawaii	12.9	6.4	14.6	14.6	13.3	2.0
Idaho	29.7	26.1	19.7	27.3	9.5	5.2
Iowa	38.1	48.1	13.5	45.0	11.9	6.0
Kansas	34.4	39.6	58.4	42.4	19.3	4.7
Maine	25.4	10.4	9.7	35.0	11.4	4.9
Massachusetts	24.5	11.2	14.6	23.0	9.6	3.5
Michigan	28.9	21.4	28.2	35.7	18.7	4.7
Mississippi	55.3	66.9	28.5	59.3	47.3	19.9
Missouri	31.5	47.1	36.4	39.5	18.7	8.5
Montana	32.4	31.5	71.8	34.2	19.8	8.2
Nebraska	30.1	50.0	33.5	45.4	14.9	7.8
New Hampshire	30.7	22.2	9.3	26.9	12.8	7.0
New York†	44.5	22.8	9.6	40.3	26.6	7.6
North Carolina	31.4	21.1	62.0	45.9	15.8	8.2
North Dakota	41.2	44.8	24.5	52.6	16.8	7.8
Oregon	35.4	13.0	20.1	31.5	20.0	12.9
Pennsylvania	27.4	19.4	34.4	28.4	18.8	6.4
Rhode Island	21.7	10.3	40.5	28.7	14.1	5.0
South Carolina	32.4	21.8	49.2	33.6	14.2	6.5
South Dakota	40.1	31.3	25.4	30.0	8.4	10.4
Tennessee	36.0	28.7	45.8	47.8	19.5	10.2
Texas	45.2	34.4	26.7	39.0	16.5	9.4
Utah	31.4	42.4	9.4	43.5	9.3	6.8
Vermont	34.3	23.0	15.4	37.6	5.4	8.9
Virginia	24.2	21.9	55.8	86.3	17.5	8.9
West Virginia	36.8	31.4	27.1	49.6	24.1	10.8
State Median	**32.4**	**24.3**	**26.9**	**38.3**	**16.7**	**7.8**
State Range	**12.9 - 66.3**	**6.4 - 66.9**	**9.3 - 71.8**	**14.6 - 86.3**	**5.4-47.3**	**2.0-19.9**

TABLE 9. Percentage of All Schools That Taught Required HIV* Prevention Units or Lessons in Specific Courses, Selected U.S. Sites: School Health Profiles, Lead Health Education Teacher Surveys, 2006 *(continued)*

Site	Science	Home economics or family and consumer education	Physical education	Family life education or life skills	Special education	Social studies
LOCAL SURVEYS						
Charlotte-Mecklenburg County	26.1	15.3	55.8	34.5	21.2	9.1
Chicago	44.5	8.0	37.2	46.9	27.9	9.5
Dallas	54.0	38.8	25.0	40.0	24.5	10.4
District of Columbia	37.3	3.7	81.6	38.1	13.9	3.5
Hillsborough County	75.8	22.1	13.7	33.7	14.4	0.0
Los Angeles	53.8	8.4	6.4	28.7	56.3	4.7
Memphis	44.9	46.2	83.4	71.2	45.4	24.2
Miami	69.3	27.7	36.1	47.3	30.9	26.4
Orange County	69.1	14.3	11.3	40.6	34.9	5.8
Philadelphia	25.4	9.7	50.0	29.2	27.8	14.5
San Diego	76.4	0.0	39.2	44.3	40.7	31.5
San Francisco	65.6	6.9	30.0	38.0	32.1	13.8
Local Median	**53.9**	**12.0**	**36.7**	**39.1**	**29.4**	**10.0**
Local Range	**25.4 - 76.4**	**0.0 - 46.2**	**6.4 - 83.4**	**28.7 - 71.2**	**13.9-56.3**	**0.0-31.5**

* Human immunodeficiency virus.
† Survey did not include schools from the New York City Department of Education.

TABLE 10a. Percentage of All Schools That Taught About Choosing Healthful Foods in a Required Health Education Course During the 2005–2006 School Year, Selected U.S. Sites: School Health Profiles, Lead Health Education Teacher Surveys, 2006

Site	Benefits of healthy eating	Using food labels	Food guidance using MyPyramid*	Eating more fruits, vegetables, and grain products	Choosing foods that are low in fat, saturated fat, and cholesterol	Using sugars in moderation	Using salt and sodium in moderation	Eating more calcium-rich foods
STATE SURVEYS								
Alabama	76.0	73.0	69.6	75.1	73.3	72.5	71.7	69.0
Alaska	72.5	67.6	61.8	70.5	68.4	69.1	63.2	61.3
Arizona	42.4	37.9	35.7	41.7	40.1	39.3	36.0	37.4
Arkansas	95.9	90.7	89.5	93.7	92.8	92.2	89.8	86.2
Connecticut	83.9	76.7	72.9	81.9	81.6	80.1	77.6	73.6
Delaware	90.3	83.5	81.8	88.5	86.9	85.3	83.6	75.2
Florida	53.6	51.2	49.9	53.0	52.3	52.2	51.6	52.3
Georgia	88.5	84.8	82.6	87.0	86.7	85.0	85.0	79.8
Hawaii	96.1	89.0	85.2	90.3	91.6	90.8	82.8	82.0
Idaho	93.8	91.4	88.3	94.1	93.0	91.4	90.4	91.0
Iowa	72.1	66.6	63.9	69.8	67.9	65.7	65.1	65.2
Kansas	74.3	66.6	66.8	72.2	70.7	71.8	68.0	66.8
Maine	89.6	82.1	77.8	84.9	87.3	85.7	84.9	79.8
Massachusetts	79.0	71.7	70.5	77.5	75.3	73.4	69.1	70.0
Michigan	75.1	68.7	67.2	74.2	72.5	71.1	68.1	65.3
Mississippi	97.9	95.0	89.7	96.6	95.4	94.7	92.9	92.4
Missouri	85.5	82.1	80.9	84.4	83.8	81.6	80.8	81.1
Montana	93.4	84.5	86.2	91.6	90.9	90.9	87.3	87.4
Nebraska	81.9	70.8	72.1	77.8	78.6	72.6	71.1	70.7
New Hampshire	81.7	78.8	77.8	79.9	79.3	79.4	77.8	75.9
New York†	98.2	89.1	86.5	97.0	96.7	94.5	92.1	90.1
North Carolina	85.7	83.4	78.6	84.8	84.2	82.8	81.0	80.1
North Dakota	87.7	80.0	81.7	84.4	80.1	80.5	80.4	81.3
Oregon	91.4	85.3	82.0	89.6	89.5	89.6	84.7	80.9
Pennsylvania	89.8	82.6	82.1	87.6	87.5	85.6	82.8	79.4
Rhode Island	93.0	87.0	84.7	90.7	91.8	84.6	82.2	84.3
South Carolina	68.1	61.8	62.3	68.1	66.2	63.7	62.5	60.1
South Dakota	65.4	56.1	57.0	61.9	60.2	59.2	56.1	54.5
Tennessee	68.0	62.5	59.8	66.5	65.7	63.2	62.5	61.1
Texas	77.8	74.4	72.6	76.1	75.3	74.1	73.4	72.3
Utah	94.7	90.4	90.2	94.2	92.1	90.4	87.1	87.4
Vermont	78.8	66.4	63.4	75.7	73.2	72.9	68.7	63.7
Virginia	82.2	77.8	76.8	82.2	81.0	79.7	78.2	76.6
West Virginia	97.7	95.6	92.5	95.0	96.0	95.0	92.2	88.7
State Median	**84.7**	**79.4**	**77.8**	**83.3**	**81.3**	**80.3**	**79.3**	**76.3**
State Range	**42.4 - 98.2**	**37.9 - 95.6**	**35.7 - 92.5**	**41.7 - 97.0**	**40.1 - 96.7**	**39.3 - 95.0**	**36.0 - 92.9**	**37.4 - 92.4**

TABLE 10a. Percentage of All Schools That Taught About Choosing Healthful Foods in a Required Health Education Course During the 2005–2006 School Year, Selected U.S. Sites: School Health Profiles, Lead Health Education Teacher Surveys, 2006 *(continued)*

Site	Benefits of healthy eating	Using food labels	Food guidance using MyPyramid*	Eating more fruits, vegetables, and grain products	Choosing foods that are low in fat, saturated fat, and cholesterol	Using sugars in moderation	Using salt and sodium in moderation	Eating more calcium-rich foods
LOCAL SURVEYS								
Charlotte-Mecklenburg County	97.4	94.5	89.1	94.5	91.9	94.5	91.9	83.4
Chicago	49.6	43.8	43.6	48.3	44.9	45.0	43.6	41.6
Dallas	56.3	56.3	56.3	54.2	56.3	52.1	54.2	50.0
District of Columbia	69.1	62.1	65.8	69.1	69.1	62.4	58.8	62.4
Hillsborough County	41.0	37.4	37.1	41.0	41.0	39.2	41.0	41.0
Los Angeles	100.0	98.7	98.7	100.0	98.7	98.7	95.1	94.0
Memphis	82.2	74.5	71.6	82.2	82.2	73.3	74.2	76.4
Miami	50.0	47.5	46.3	50.0	50.0	50.0	47.5	48.8
Orange County	46.6	40.9	46.6	46.6	43.6	43.6	43.6	43.6
Philadelphia	83.5	77.3	75.5	81.6	80.5	75.3	75.2	69.1
San Diego‡	0.0	0.0	0.0	0.0	0.0	0.0	0.0	0.0
San Francisco	57.2	53.6	53.6	53.6	53.6	53.6	53.6	53.6
Local Median	**56.8**	**55.0**	**55.0**	**53.9**	**55.0**	**52.9**	**53.9**	**51.8**
Local Range	**0.0 – 100.0**	**0.0 – 98.7**	**0.0 – 98.7**	**0.0 – 100.0**	**0.0 – 98.7**	**0.0 – 98.7**	**0.0 – 95.1**	**0.0 – 94.0**

* Visit the MyPyramid Web site at http://www.mypyramid.gov.
† Survey did not include schools from the New York City Department of Education.
‡ San Diego does not have a required health education course, but requires that health education be taught in science and physical education classes.

TABLE 10b. Percentage of All Schools That Taught About Food Safety and Behaviors That Contribute to Maintaining a Healthy Weight in a Required Health Education Course During the 2005–2006 School Year, Selected U.S. Sites: School Health Profiles, Lead Health Education Teacher Surveys, 2006

Site	Food safety	Balancing food intake and physical activity	Preparing healthy meals and snacks	Risks of unhealthy weight control practices	Accepting body size differences	Eating disorders
STATE SURVEYS						
Alabama	69.2	74.4	71.8	74.1	73.8	73.9
Alaska	59.6	69.5	63.7	64.8	61.1	57.9
Arizona	33.3	41.2	36.0	38.6	37.1	36.1
Arkansas	83.7	95.6	89.2	92.4	88.9	90.5
Connecticut	59.5	80.3	65.0	80.7	76.2	76.5
Delaware	74.8	90.2	80.0	90.0	83.6	80.2
Florida	47.8	53.0	50.4	51.3	49.5	52.0
Georgia	78.4	87.4	80.7	86.2	84.8	86.3
Hawaii	73.3	94.7	82.4	87.9	85.8	85.3
Idaho	82.6	94.1	84.4	93.0	90.4	91.3
Iowa	58.5	70.9	58.9	69.5	64.1	69.3
Kansas	60.6	73.2	62.2	70.2	70.0	71.6
Maine	68.2	87.8	73.0	83.8	82.0	80.6
Massachusetts	57.3	77.2	63.6	74.3	74.4	74.2
Michigan	58.4	73.9	66.4	72.7	69.3	66.7
Mississippi	93.1	97.3	93.5	96.7	94.4	94.4
Missouri	75.6	84.5	77.8	82.2	79.4	81.8
Montana	79.2	93.9	83.9	92.5	89.7	92.0
Nebraska	67.5	81.9	68.1	81.0	76.4	76.5
New Hampshire	66.8	79.7	69.3	78.2	77.3	76.7
New York*	76.0	96.5	87.6	97.3	94.1	95.2
North Carolina	75.1	85.6	81.7	84.4	81.4	82.6
North Dakota	77.5	84.3	77.3	82.4	79.9	81.7
Oregon	73.7	90.5	80.0	87.3	87.3	87.4
Pennsylvania	68.7	90.1	80.1	87.7	84.7	85.9
Rhode Island	77.2	89.5	78.5	95.4	89.3	93.0
South Carolina	56.8	67.4	60.6	65.1	62.3	63.2
South Dakota	48.4	61.3	51.8	55.7	54.6	58.3
Tennessee	58.5	66.4	61.9	66.7	60.2	62.8
Texas	69.9	76.2	74.5	75.9	74.6	74.7
Utah	75.2	92.6	80.7	92.2	92.0	93.6
Vermont	52.7	73.9	61.1	69.2	68.9	67.6
Virginia	70.1	81.2	73.9	78.5	73.1	76.3
West Virginia	84.9	96.1	93.4	94.3	93.9	95.4
State Median	**69.6**	**83.1**	**74.2**	**81.6**	**78.4**	**78.5**
State Range	**33.3 – 93.1**	**41.2 – 97.3**	**36.0 – 93.5**	**38.6 – 97.3**	**37.1 – 94.4**	**36.1 – 95.4**

TABLE 10b. Percentage of All Schools That Taught About Food Safety and Behaviors That Contribute to Maintaining a Healthy Weight in a Required Health Education Course During the 2005–2006 School Year, Selected U.S. Sites: School Health Profiles, Lead Health Education Teacher Surveys, 2006 *(continued)*

Site	Food safety	Balancing food intake and physical activity	Preparing healthy meals and snacks	Risks of unhealthy weight control practices	Accepting body size difference	Eating disorders
LOCAL SURVEYS						
Charlotte-Mecklenburg County	65.2	94.7	94.7	97.4	91.9	89.3
Chicago	39.4	48.8	43.9	43.4	45.0	39.8
Dallas	52.1	54.2	47.9	54.2	54.2	56.3
District of Columbia	58.5	67.9	65.8	61.0	62.1	55.5
Hillsborough County	34.4	41.0	38.9	41.0	40.3	41.0
Los Angeles	89.2	100.0	91.5	98.7	93.9	95.0
Memphis	76.2	82.2	72.9	80.6	71.8	74.7
Miami	47.5	50.0	48.7	48.8	48.7	48.1
Orange County	40.9	46.6	43.6	43.6	43.6	43.6
Philadelphia	71.7	81.6	80.5	76.9	72.1	73.0
San Diego†	0.0	0.0	0.0	0.0	0.0	0.0
San Francisco	42.9	50.0	53.6	53.6	57.2	57.2
Local Median	**49.8**	**52.1**	**51.2**	**53.9**	**55.7**	**55.9**
Local Range	**0.0 - 89.2**	**0.0 - 100.0**	**0.0 - 94.7**	**0.0 - 98.7**	**0.0 - 93.9**	**0.0 - 95.0**

* Survey did not include schools from the New York City Department of Education.

† San Diego does not have a required health education course, but requires that health education be taught in science and physical education classes.

TABLE 11a. Percentage of All Schools That Taught About the Benefits of Physical Activity and Guidance for Engaging in Physical Activity in a Required Health Education Course During the 2005–2006 School Year, Selected U.S. Sites: School Health Profiles, Lead Health Education Teacher Surveys, 2006

Site	Physical, psychological, or social benefits	Health-related fitness	Difference between physical activity, exercise, and fitness	Phases of a workout	How much physical activity is enough	Decreasing sedentary activities
STATE SURVEYS						
Alabama	76.2	74.5	72.1	73.4	72.3	74.2
Alaska	70.3	65.9	55.8	62.3	59.3	60.7
Arizona	41.4	41.3	36.8	36.8	35.1	40.2
Arkansas	94.8	93.8	90.8	91.8	90.1	91.2
Connecticut	77.7	67.2	57.8	58.5	60.0	68.6
Delaware	86.9	85.3	80.2	80.1	78.9	86.9
Florida	51.4	47.8	45.6	43.8	44.1	48.6
Georgia	86.7	85.1	81.4	80.4	80.9	82.7
Hawaii	90.8	79.3	70.7	71.4	72.9	81.2
Idaho	92.6	88.3	82.0	84.6	86.2	88.7
Iowa	71.1	70.0	66.5	61.1	61.5	66.1
Kansas	72.1	72.6	66.3	67.9	67.9	67.5
Maine	82.8	76.0	67.4	68.5	67.3	75.0
Massachusetts	76.7	67.3	58.2	58.1	58.7	69.4
Michigan	74.0	68.6	63.3	64.0	64.4	65.6
Mississippi	95.5	91.7	86.6	84.2	84.0	90.9
Missouri	83.2	80.9	77.2	77.6	77.8	79.4
Montana	94.4	93.1	88.3	93.2	88.1	90.9
Nebraska	81.5	77.0	72.1	73.5	73.7	73.4
New Hampshire	79.9	71.1	56.9	57.8	62.5	73.5
New York*	94.9	85.5	75.3	68.5	79.3	92.0
North Carolina	86.5	85.2	77.8	82.3	76.4	83.2
North Dakota	87.3	83.7	79.1	80.1	74.3	82.9
Oregon	90.3	84.2	78.1	79.2	79.1	82.8
Pennsylvania	89.9	87.6	78.9	82.4	79.0	86.4
Rhode Island	91.6	85.8	83.1	83.4	83.5	83.4
South Carolina	67.3	65.2	61.8	63.4	62.2	63.0
South Dakota	66.0	65.0	58.5	56.7	54.9	61.1
Tennessee	68.5	68.2	64.6	67.2	64.5	66.6
Texas	76.3	76.7	74.5	68.6	71.1	74.1
Utah	92.9	88.7	82.9	80.4	81.5	88.0
Vermont	69.3	59.3	49.0	48.4	55.5	60.5
Virginia	82.4	81.3	75.0	76.9	77.5	79.3
West Virginia	96.7	94.5	86.8	90.0	92.2	93.6
State Median	**82.6**	**78.2**	**73.3**	**72.4**	**73.3**	**77.2**
State Range	**41.4 - 96.7**	**41.3 - 94.5**	**36.8 - 90.8**	**36.8 - 93.2**	**35.1 - 92.2**	**40.2 - 93.6**

TABLE 11a. Percentage of All Schools That Taught About the Benefits of Physical Activity and Guidance for Engaging in Physical Activity in a Required Health Education Course During the 2005–2006 School Year, Selected U.S. Sites: School Health Profiles, Lead Health Education Teacher Surveys, 2006 *(continued)*

Site	Physical, psychological, or social benefits	Health-related fitness	Difference between physical activity, exercise, and fitness	Phases of a workout	How much physical activity is enough	Decreasing sedentary activities
LOCAL SURVEYS						
Charlotte-Mecklenburg County	91.6	86.0	72.1	83.1	85.8	91.4
Chicago	50.8	47.4	44.4	45.2	41.3	45.0
Dallas	51.1	45.7	45.8	39.6	37.5	46.8
District of Columbia	72.1	75.5	64.3	75.5	63.6	68.3
Hillsborough County	39.1	38.0	35.9	32.1	32.8	37.2
Los Angeles	92.6	90.1	80.5	77.4	86.8	92.8
Memphis	84.6	84.6	81.1	84.6	82.8	82.2
Miami	47.5	41.8	38.5	38.5	40.5	45.6
Orange County	41.9	35.6	30.6	38.3	33.5	39.1
Philadelphia	76.6	76.6	69.7	74.4	65.8	65.4
San Diego†	0.0	0.0	0.0	0.0	0.0	0.0
San Francisco	53.6	53.6	50.0	46.4	50.0	53.6
Local Median	**52.4**	**50.5**	**47.9**	**45.8**	**45.7**	**50.2**
Local Range	**0.0 – 92.6**	**0.0 – 90.1**	**0.0 – 81.1**	**0.0 – 84.6**	**0.0 – 86.8**	**0.0 – 92.8**

* Survey did not include schools from the New York City Department of Education.

† San Diego does not have a required health education course, but requires that health education be taught in science and physical education classes.

TABLE 11b. Percentage of All Schools That Taught About the Challenges to Engaging in Physical Activity in a Required Health Education Course During the 2005–2006 School Year, Selected U.S. Sites: School Health Profiles, Lead Health Education Teacher Surveys, 2006

Site	Overcoming barriers to physical activity	Developing an individualized physical activity plan	Monitoring progress toward reaching goals	Opportunities for physical activity in the community	Preventing injury during physical activity	Weather-related safety	Dangers of using performance-enhancing drugs
STATE SURVEYS							
Alabama	67.6	63.4	64.3	69.8	74.0	72.0	75.0
Alaska	52.4	49.7	48.3	59.4	57.6	56.0	58.2
Arizona	32.6	29.1	28.9	33.0	36.3	37.4	34.3
Arkansas	79.3	79.6	74.8	81.8	92.8	89.1	92.4
Connecticut	54.5	49.0	48.7	61.2	63.0	55.2	77.9
Delaware	78.6	65.3	66.3	81.9	81.8	73.6	83.4
Florida	43.9	39.5	38.1	41.7	44.0	47.0	47.3
Georgia	77.2	72.4	72.4	78.3	84.8	83.7	86.0
Hawaii	70.2	67.0	61.6	74.8	68.0	74.2	87.3
Idaho	75.2	76.1	67.2	75.8	85.0	82.9	89.4
Iowa	55.5	51.7	48.4	56.0	61.0	61.1	68.2
Kansas	54.9	50.8	47.9	54.1	64.9	63.2	71.2
Maine	61.4	61.0	55.1	64.7	70.6	68.3	76.6
Massachusetts	52.3	46.6	45.1	56.0	59.6	60.5	72.3
Michigan	58.0	54.2	49.9	56.4	62.0	58.7	69.0
Mississippi	77.4	67.2	63.9	81.9	87.9	88.9	95.3
Missouri	67.2	65.9	60.6	68.0	77.3	76.9	79.9
Montana	81.4	70.6	68.6	79.7	92.4	84.4	89.0
Nebraska	59.6	57.2	54.4	64.1	71.7	70.6	80.9
New Hampshire	59.6	52.2	49.8	63.2	63.8	65.6	76.9
New York*	73.4	55.9	50.0	73.0	73.8	80.4	96.3
North Carolina	73.2	71.1	69.6	79.3	81.9	77.4	81.6
North Dakota	69.2	58.3	50.4	70.5	74.9	76.0	83.6
Oregon	68.5	66.4	60.1	70.6	77.9	70.5	83.1
Pennsylvania	69.4	66.2	64.2	73.3	80.7	73.7	83.5
Rhode Island	76.2	59.7	59.6	73.6	79.7	71.2	88.0
South Carolina	60.0	54.5	51.7	62.5	64.3	59.2	64.3
South Dakota	48.6	41.7	40.5	52.0	59.4	50.6	58.3
Tennessee	57.7	53.0	51.4	57.5	66.6	59.2	62.6
Texas	64.4	63.6	59.8	66.2	72.0	72.6	75.4
Utah	74.3	68.1	64.2	74.4	80.8	75.2	89.7
Vermont	46.4	41.7	41.6	52.1	49.7	49.8	65.3
Virginia	70.1	67.9	66.7	70.6	76.7	72.0	77.2
West Virginia	84.2	74.7	70.9	85.9	92.9	89.3	92.7
State Median	**67.4**	**60.4**	**57.4**	**68.9**	**72.9**	**71.6**	**78.9**
State Range	**32.6 - 84.2**	**29.1 - 79.6**	**28.9 - 74.8**	**33.0 - 85.9**	**36.3 - 92.9**	**37.4 - 89.3**	**34.3 - 96.3**

TABLE 11b. Percentage of All Schools That Taught About the Challenges to Engaging in Physical Activity in a Required Health Education Course During the 2005–2006 School Year, Selected U.S. Sites: School Health Profiles, Lead Health Education Teacher Surveys, 2006 *(continued)*

Site	Overcoming barriers to physical activity	Developing an individualized physical activity plan	Monitoring progress toward reaching goals	Opportunities for physical activity in the community	Preventing injury during physical activity	Weather-related safety	Dangers of using performance-enhancing drugs
LOCAL SURVEYS							
Charlotte-Mecklenburg County	69.4	69.6	69.4	80.0	82.9	74.0	88.8
Chicago	41.0	33.1	32.7	37.9	47.4	41.3	41.4
Dallas	37.5	33.3	31.3	44.7	41.7	45.7	52.2
District of Columbia	65.7	61.4	63.3	68.3	72.1	61.1	57.7
Hillsborough County	29.5	28.8	26.7	24.6	32.1	34.9	37.0
Los Angeles	80.6	77.0	69.8	72.1	78.3	79.1	94.8
Memphis	79.5	79.3	79.5	77.1	84.6	78.0	80.4
Miami	43.6	39.8	37.2	42.4	41.1	43.7	45.5
Orange County	33.6	30.0	36.4	29.7	33.9	44.9	43.2
Philadelphia	61.6	61.4	59.1	63.6	69.4	59.3	64.7
San Diego†	0.0	0.0	0.0	0.0	0.0	0.0	0.0
San Francisco	50.0	42.9	39.3	35.7	46.4	48.2	57.2
Local Median	**46.8**	**41.4**	**38.3**	**43.6**	**46.9**	**47.0**	**54.7**
Local Range	**0.0 – 80.6**	**0.0 – 79.3**	**0.0 – 79.5**	**0.0 – 80.0**	**0.0 – 84.6**	**0.0 – 79.1**	**0.0 – 94.8**

* Survey did not include schools from the New York City Department of Education.

† San Diego does not have a required health education course, but requires that health education be taught in science and physical education classes.

TABLE 12. Percentage of All Schools That Taught All 16 Tobacco-Use Prevention Topics; All 11 Pregnancy, HIV* or STD† Prevention Topics; All 14 Nutrition and Dietary Behavior Topics; or All 13 Physical Activity Topics in a Required Health Education Course During the 2005–2006 School Year, Selected U.S. Sites: School Health Profiles, Lead Health Education Teacher Surveys, 2006

Site	Taught all 16 tobacco-use prevention topics	Taught all 11 pregnancy, HIV, or STD prevention topics	Taught all 14 nutrition and dietary behavior topics	Taught all 13 physical activity topics
STATE SURVEYS				
Alabama	58.1	21.0	57.0	54.2
Alaska	32.8	18.8	42.9	27.9
Arizona	23.1	9.0	23.8	20.1
Arkansas	66.3	19.1	71.8	62.0
Connecticut	43.7	32.6	45.9	24.8
Delaware	51.9	37.8	59.6	56.3
Florida	35.0	21.2	40.2	28.2
Georgia	64.8	18.3	67.2	60.1
Hawaii	50.0	44.9	60.0	37.6
Idaho	58.6	16.1	69.1	52.0
Iowa	37.7	23.7	43.2	35.8
Kansas	34.4	15.2	44.3	31.6
Maine	39.3	34.9	53.1	39.4
Massachusetts	41.9	30.8	45.3	31.5
Michigan	37.6	19.7	43.8	32.5
Mississippi	70.8	28.5	78.0	52.1
Missouri	51.1	16.8	64.8	46.6
Montana	59.2	26.5	64.5	54.8
Nebraska	44.4	16.8	52.5	37.4
New Hampshire	47.6	37.4	56.2	37.9
New York‡	67.8	53.1	64.5	34.4
North Carolina	58.5	12.1	66.0	52.8
North Dakota	51.9	15.3	65.7	40.8
Oregon	42.2	35.0	54.6	39.8
Pennsylvania	56.2	29.7	57.7	44.1
Rhode Island	59.6	39.9	63.5	45.3
South Carolina	43.0	23.0	46.5	42.7
South Dakota	34.5	9.5	35.7	27.5
Tennessee	39.4	15.5	46.0	39.0
Texas	50.5	15.1	61.3	48.8
Utah	51.5	1.0	63.1	43.4
Vermont	30.8	33.3	40.5	25.4
Virginia	48.6	1.5	58.8	50.2
West Virginia	74.5	31.0	75.9	58.2
State Median	**49.3**	**21.1**	**57.4**	**40.3**
State Range	**23.1 – 74.5**	**1.0 – 53.1**	**23.8 – 78.0**	**20.1 – 62.0**

TABLE 12. Percentage of All Schools That Taught All 16 Tobacco-Use Prevention Topics; All 11 Pregnancy, HIV* or STD† Prevention Topics; All 14 Nutrition and Dietary Behavior Topics; or All 13 Physical Activity Topics in a Required Health Education Course During the 2005–2006 School Year, Selected U.S. Sites: School Health Profiles, Lead Health Education Teacher Surveys, 2006 *(continued)*

Site	Taught all 16 tobacco-use prevention topics	Taught all 11 pregnancy, HIV, or STD prevention topics	Taught all 14 nutrition and dietary behavior topics	Taught all 13 physical activity topics
LOCAL SURVEYS				
Charlotte-Mecklenburg County	59.5	13.9	59.7	50.2
Chicago	23.0	16.8	28.8	22.3
Dallas	38.3	10.4	43.8	22.9
District of Columbia	38.5	44.0	48.5	36.0
Hillsborough County	33.0	18.2	30.6	20.0
Los Angeles	76.8	66.5	79.2	50.9
Memphis	51.1	33.7	56.0	64.8
Miami	37.9	40.0	39.9	33.8
Orange County	33.2	32.0	40.9	24.3
Philadelphia	44.8	28.5	55.1	33.8
San Diego§	0.0	0.0	0.0	0.0
San Francisco	32.1	28.6	42.9	28.6
Local Median	**38.1**	**28.6**	**43.4**	**31.2**
Local Range	**0.0 - 76.8**	**0.0 - 66.5**	**0.0 - 79.2**	**0.0 - 64.8**

* Human immunodeficiency virus.
† Sexually transmitted disease.
‡ Survey did not include schools from the New York City Department of Education.
§ San Diego does not have a required health education course, but requires that health education be taught in science and physical education classes.

TABLE 13a. Percentage of All Schools That Sometimes, Almost Always, or Always Used Specific Teaching Methods in a Required Health Education Course During the 2005–2006 School Year, Selected U.S. Sites: School Health Profiles, Lead Health Education Teacher Surveys, 2006

Site	Audio-visual media, (e.g., videos)	Group discussions	Cooperative group activities	Role play simulations, or practice	Language, performing, or visual arts	Pledges or contracts for changing behavior or abstaining from a behavior
STATE SURVEYS						
Alabama	74.1	76.8	70.6	49.2	35.2	40.1
Alaska	59.8	72.0	65.6	46.1	35.7	23.0
Arizona	39.1	42.6	39.9	32.0	23.0	21.9
Arkansas	83.1	95.6	84.5	53.2	35.4	29.5
Connecticut	79.3	86.8	84.3	65.1	42.6	22.7
Delaware	82.5	92.0	91.8	73.1	45.2	29.8
Florida	49.9	53.4	50.1	39.2	29.7	25.0
Georgia	85.3	87.4	81.1	68.1	49.4	41.3
Hawaii	77.5	96.1	90.5	78.5	66.1	43.3
Idaho	86.7	92.7	85.7	57.7	42.2	30.3
Iowa	66.2	72.1	68.4	47.3	34.8	19.0
Kansas	64.5	73.6	68.5	42.4	30.0	18.7
Maine	80.7	91.2	86.4	65.9	42.6	21.3
Massachusetts	78.4	82.4	80.2	64.3	44.6	24.2
Michigan	72.7	77.9	75.6	54.6	37.9	24.6
Mississippi	90.8	94.1	87.2	60.5	46.1	31.9
Missouri	78.5	84.6	77.6	52.4	40.5	32.5
Montana	87.1	95.2	88.2	55.0	36.6	24.8
Nebraska	81.1	84.5	78.5	49.4	39.1	26.5
New Hampshire	74.5	83.3	80.1	66.7	44.1	20.0
New York*	92.8	97.8	94.3	78.0	55.6	36.7
North Carolina	80.1	84.7	80.1	60.1	44.7	35.3
North Dakota	83.0	88.4	83.6	61.6	45.7	26.9
Oregon	85.9	93.8	91.7	67.9	51.8	27.8
Pennsylvania	89.1	92.4	87.1	59.8	41.4	27.7
Rhode Island	84.6	95.4	90.7	71.3	51.5	31.4
South Carolina	66.0	71.1	65.6	51.7	37.7	38.7
South Dakota	58.9	67.6	63.0	40.3	28.5	17.5
Tennessee	61.8	70.0	64.1	40.0	33.5	31.2
Texas	70.2	76.7	72.6	45.4	37.4	29.5
Utah	89.4	94.3	88.3	65.0	48.4	32.9
Vermont	71.9	80.4	77.0	61.0	38.7	19.9
Virginia	78.9	82.0	76.8	53.9	39.0	29.1
West Virginia	91.7	97.3	90.7	61.9	53.8	34.6
State Median	**79.1**	**84.7**	**80.2**	**58.8**	**41.0**	**28.5**
State Range	**39.1 – 92.8**	**42.6 – 97.8**	**39.9 – 94.3**	**32.0 – 78.5**	**23.0 – 66.1**	**17.5 – 43.3**

TABLE 13a. Percentage of All Schools That Sometimes, Almost Always, or Always Used Specific Teaching Methods in a Required Health Education Course During the 2005–2006 School Year, Selected U.S. Sites: School Health Profiles, Lead Health Education Teacher Surveys, 2006 *(continued)*

Site	Audio-visual media, (e.g., videos)	Group discussions	Cooperative group activities	Role play simulations, or practice	Language, performing, or visual arts	Pledges or contracts for changing behavior or abstaining from a behavior
LOCAL SURVEYS						
Charlotte-Mecklenburg County	86.4	100.0	94.7	83.8	66.7	49.0
Chicago	46.5	51.2	48.8	37.0	33.6	31.6
Dallas	56.3	56.3	52.1	37.5	39.6	18.8
District of Columbia	62.4	76.4	69.1	62.4	48.4	42.8
Hillsborough County	43.7	44.7	40.7	30.9	23.8	16.7
Los Angeles	94.9	95.0	97.7	81.1	76.1	54.8
Memphis	76.4	84.6	80.6	68.3	63.5	38.7
Miami	44.8	51.3	46.1	37.6	32.0	24.3
Orange County	49.5	49.5	49.5	32.9	24.3	16.6
Philadelphia	75.8	83.7	80.7	56.1	49.7	39.1
San Diego†	0.0	0.0	0.0	0.0	0.0	0.0
San Francisco	50.0	53.6	53.6	48.2	48.2	17.8
Local Median	**53.2**	**55.0**	**52.9**	**42.9**	**43.9**	**28.0**
Local Range	**0.0 - 94.9**	**0.0 - 100.0**	**0.0 - 97.7**	**0.0 - 83.8**	**0.0 - 76.1**	**0.0 - 54.8**

* Survey did not include schools from the New York City Department of Education.

† San Diego does not have a required health education course, but requires that health education be taught in science and physical education classes.

TABLE 13b. Percentage of All Schools That Sometimes, Almost Always, or Always Used Specific Teaching Methods in a Required Health Education Course During the 2005–2006 School Year, Selected U.S. Sites: School Health Profiles, Lead Health Education Teacher Surveys, 2006

Site	Peer teaching	Internet	Computer-assisted instruction	Guest speakers	Health education programs through available distance learning methods
STATE SURVEYS					
Alabama	47.8	58.6	40.5	57.8	14.9
Alaska	49.4	64.4	37.9	49.1	14.0
Arizona	28.7	31.5	22.5	29.8	5.0
Arkansas	51.3	61.2	37.3	51.8	9.9
Connecticut	54.0	70.7	48.7	51.0	5.4
Delaware	61.1	68.0	41.8	66.5	1.7
Florida	32.2	40.3	25.3	42.6	9.0
Georgia	56.5	67.0	51.5	54.7	12.3
Hawaii	82.7	70.5	41.6	77.2	5.3
Idaho	61.3	71.3	44.5	61.4	5.6
Iowa	46.4	58.3	37.3	45.0	8.5
Kansas	43.6	57.3	37.8	36.8	7.0
Maine	48.6	79.6	53.0	56.9	3.6
Massachusetts	48.1	60.6	39.6	44.6	4.8
Michigan	42.8	55.4	37.3	47.0	6.9
Mississippi	57.5	75.9	57.3	62.4	16.7
Missouri	49.9	64.2	44.3	53.0	10.2
Montana	55.2	68.0	51.0	67.2	8.9
Nebraska	44.4	64.5	42.1	48.6	6.0
New Hampshire	49.6	62.1	36.6	52.7	5.9
New York*	63.5	85.4	62.4	69.6	5.9
North Carolina	54.3	58.5	39.5	59.0	9.8
North Dakota	54.3	79.4	52.0	52.9	7.5
Oregon	61.9	73.3	42.5	59.0	8.8
Pennsylvania	50.1	70.6	42.9	57.9	5.9
Rhode Island	54.9	73.6	53.8	60.2	9.8
South Carolina	44.0	48.6	34.8	41.7	8.7
South Dakota	36.0	58.7	40.1	36.2	7.1
Tennessee	40.1	48.7	36.1	54.6	9.5
Texas	53.3	55.1	43.7	41.1	10.6
Utah	57.7	61.0	39.3	72.7	8.0
Vermont	46.4	53.2	33.6	49.7	3.5
Virginia	48.2	64.4	54.1	47.0	6.5
West Virginia	58.1	76.3	59.1	66.4	14.8
State Median	**50.0**	**64.3**	**41.7**	**53.0**	**7.8**
State Range	**28.7 - 82.7**	**31.5 - 85.4**	**22.5 - 62.4**	**29.8 - 77.2**	**1.7 - 16.7**

TABLE 13b. Percentage of All Schools That Sometimes, Almost Always, or Always Used Specific Teaching Methods in a Required Health Education Course During the 2005–2006 School Year, Selected U.S. Sites: School Health Profiles, Lead Health Education Teacher Surveys, 2006 *(continued)*

Site	Peer teaching	Internet	Computer-assisted instruction	Guest speakers	Health education programs through available distance learning methods
LOCAL SURVEYS					
Charlotte-Mecklenburg County	55.7	51.6	40.7	64.8	10.7
Chicago	33.1	39.5	27.4	35.5	9.6
Dallas	41.7	35.4	27.1	38.3	10.4
District of Columbia	45.1	42.1	36.4	62.0	14.2
Hillsborough County	21.6	25.7	9.8	44.0	3.4
Los Angeles	75.2	82.9	59.1	64.7	12.1
Memphis	63.5	72.1	48.9	57.2	23.5
Miami	34.6	39.8	20.5	41.5	6.4
Orange County	27.9	38.6	14.0	35.9	2.7
Philadelphia	48.9	46.7	30.4	38.0	10.4
San Diego†	0.0	0.0	0.0	0.0	0.0
San Francisco	42.9	37.1	14.3	46.5	0.0
Local Median	**42.3**	**39.7**	**27.3**	**42.8**	**10.0**
Local Range	**0.0 - 75.2**	**0.0 - 82.9**	**0.0 - 59.1**	**0.0 - 64.8**	**0.0 - 23.5**

* Survey did not include schools from the New York City Department of Education.

† San Diego does not have a required health education course, but requires that health education be taught in science and physical education classes.

TABLE 14. Percentage of All Schools That Used Specific Methods to Highlight Diversity or the Values of Various Cultures in a Required Health Education Course During the 2005–2006 School Year, Selected U.S. Sites: School Health Profiles, Lead Health Education Teacher Surveys, 2006

Site	Using textbooks or curricular materials reflective of various cultures	Using textbooks or curricular materials designed for students with limited English proficiency	Asking students or families to share their own cultural experiences related to health topics	Teaching about cultural differences and similarities	Modifying teaching methods to match students' learning styles, health beliefs, or cultural values
STATE SURVEYS					
Alabama	54.8	26.2	55.7	64.1	69.8
Alaska	53.6	21.8	54.3	63.2	68.1
Arizona	31.2	21.6	32.4	36.4	40.6
Arkansas	64.7	34.1	61.0	82.6	85.2
Connecticut	46.9	16.9	53.3	61.3	81.3
Delaware	64.6	30.4	57.8	74.6	88.6
Florida	41.8	29.1	37.5	42.6	51.1
Georgia	57.0	30.5	63.6	72.6	80.6
Hawaii	49.7	28.4	72.3	78.7	89.3
Idaho	63.7	32.5	62.4	78.7	83.9
Iowa	53.4	18.4	43.2	57.7	66.8
Kansas	40.6	15.0	34.2	52.1	53.2
Maine	44.4	13.5	50.8	62.8	79.2
Massachusetts	50.8	18.7	54.3	64.9	73.2
Michigan	50.5	15.4	41.2	52.9	67.8
Mississippi	72.2	26.2	68.1	84.4	87.7
Missouri	58.1	22.5	48.0	67.2	72.8
Montana	54.2	11.2	57.8	75.3	79.7
Nebraska	66.1	20.5	54.5	65.6	75.1
New Hampshire	51.0	11.8	48.9	62.6	75.4
New York*	61.5	21.2	69.5	77.6	87.9
North Carolina	56.7	38.2	55.4	69.0	79.7
North Dakota	60.9	15.7	54.8	71.3	73.4
Oregon	65.5	35.9	57.8	76.1	86.1
Pennsylvania	53.3	17.3	56.2	66.0	82.1
Rhode Island	48.3	25.9	63.8	69.5	84.2
South Carolina	48.4	22.9	47.1	54.0	63.1
South Dakota	31.1	4.7	27.7	38.8	49.1
Tennessee	48.3	20.8	41.9	56.5	59.7
Texas	60.5	40.6	54.2	65.6	72.0
Utah	61.5	41.3	48.2	73.8	84.1
Vermont	42.4	9.4	37.7	53.3	74.7
Virginia	44.8	27.0	45.6	60.3	73.1
West Virginia	72.8	26.5	67.4	85.5	92.1
State Median	**53.5**	**22.2**	**54.3**	**65.6**	**75.3**
State Range	**31.1 - 72.8**	**4.7 - 41.3**	**27.7 - 72.3**	**36.4 - 85.5**	**40.6 - 92.1**

TABLE 14. Percentage of All Schools That Used Specific Methods to Highlight Diversity or the Values of Various Cultures in a Required Health Education Course During the 2005–2006 School Year, Selected U.S. Sites: School Health Profiles, Lead Health Education Teacher Surveys, 2006 *(continued)*

Site	Using textbooks or curricular materials reflective of various cultures	Using textbooks or curricular materials designed for students with limited English proficiency	Asking students or families to share their own cultural experiences related to health topics	Teaching about cultural differences and similarities	Modifying teaching methods to match students' learning styles, health beliefs, or cultural values
LOCAL SURVEYS					
Charlotte-Mecklenburg County	65.2	44.4	67.8	84.0	91.9
Chicago	37.6	21.6	37.1	47.0	47.0
Dallas	47.9	31.3	45.8	54.2	56.3
District of Columbia	45.1	20.6	55.8	59.1	66.1
Hillsborough County	31.7	25.7	25.9	37.3	41.0
Los Angeles	87.6	85.4	86.7	91.5	97.5
Memphis	62.4	43.0	63.5	73.2	78.7
Miami	39.7	33.8	39.8	46.1	44.8
Orange County	35.6	24.9	43.9	43.9	49.5
Philadelphia	59.6	19.6	51.3	67.2	71.6
San Diego†	0.0	0.0	0.0	0.0	0.0
San Francisco	46.5	28.6	35.7	53.6	55.6
Local Median	**45.8**	**27.2**	**44.9**	**53.9**	**56.0**
Local Range	**0.0 - 87.6**	**0.0 - 85.4**	**0.0 - 86.7**	**0.0 - 91.5**	**0.0 - 97.5**

* Survey did not include schools from the New York City Department of Education.
† San Diego does not have a required health education course, but requires that health education be taught in science and physical education classes.

Table 15. Percentage of All Schools with a Health Education Coordinator and, Among those Schools, the Percentage in Which Specific Staff Served as the Health Education Coordinator, Selected U.S. Sites: School Health Profiles, Principal Surveys, 2006

Site	Had a health education coordinator	District administrator or district health education or curriculum coordinator	School administrator	Health education teacher	School nurse	Someone else
STATE SURVEYS						
Alabama	95.8	21.6	33.9	37.2	2.7	4.6
Alaska	89.4	34.7	31.7	25.0	2.5	6.1
Arizona	80.4	21.8	30.6	24.8	8.6	14.2
Arkansas	96.8	16.8	27.4	53.6	0.9	1.4
Connecticut	94.3	47.1	16.6	29.6	3.5	3.2
Delaware	98.5	19.7	27.3	49.9	1.5	1.5
Florida	89.6	24.6	29.0	29.9	3.7	12.8
Georgia	98.1	24.5	23.8	48.6	0.4	2.7
Hawaii	93.2	5.9	15.4	75.1	0.0	3.7
Idaho	98.4	27.9	12.4	57.1	0.0	2.6
Illinois	98.3	19.9	20.7	55.1	0.6	3.7
Iowa	93.7	29.2	16.5	46.9	2.0	5.4
Kansas	93.2	28.3	13.4	48.6	2.6	7.1
Maine	94.9	37.6	11.0	43.1	3.9	4.5
Massachusetts	94.7	49.0	14.3	29.3	2.5	4.9
Michigan	95.1	38.0	21.1	34.6	1.8	4.5
Mississippi	94.6	16.1	32.8	45.3	4.5	1.3
Missouri	96.6	27.4	16.6	46.9	5.3	3.9
Montana	99.2	19.1	15.8	62.8	0.0	2.3
Nebraska	95.9	26.8	21.4	47.3	2.4	2.2
New Hampshire	93.0	18.0	23.4	44.2	6.9	7.5
New York*	98.1	47.5	18.5	31.9	0.0	2.2
North Carolina	97.5	24.8	14.7	56.2	0.4	3.9
North Dakota	95.8	13.4	26.9	54.5	2.2	2.9
Oregon	95.8	18.2	20.8	54.3	0.0	6.7
Pennsylvania	97.2	34.4	20.3	41.6	1.5	2.2
Rhode Island	96.3	31.9	8.5	46.2	2.4	11.0
South Carolina	96.1	27.8	19.8	46.2	1.3	4.9
South Dakota	87.4	21.7	23.7	51.7	0.0	2.8
Tennessee	91.7	28.1	22.3	37.0	5.6	7.0
Texas	93.7	26.4	25.0	41.6	5.3	1.7
Utah	99.5	19.2	18.1	59.8	1.0	1.9
Vermont	91.1	11.2	21.4	49.0	8.7	9.7
Virginia	98.3	39.1	14.9	43.5	0.7	1.8
Washington	92.8	25.6	14.7	51.4	3.4	4.9
West Virginia	97.4	10.5	28.1	60.4	0.0	1.1
State Median	**95.8**	**25.2**	**20.8**	**46.9**	**2.1**	**3.8**
State Range	**80.4 - 99.5**	**5.9 - 49.0**	**8.5 - 33.9**	**24.8 - 75.1**	**0.0 - 8.7**	**1.1 - 14.2**

Table 15. Percentage of All Schools with a Health Education Coordinator and, Among those Schools, the Percentage in Which Specific Staff Served as the Health Education Coordinator, Selected U.S. Sites: School Health Profiles, Principal Surveys, 2006 *(continued)*

Site	Had a health education coordinator	District administrator or district health education or curriculum coordinator	School administrator	Health education teacher	School nurse	Someone else
LOCAL SURVEYS						
Charlotte-Mecklenburg County	100.0	33.5	9.7	56.8	0.0	0.0
Chicago	81.4	5.8	14.3	44.8	9.1	25.9
Dallas	74.5	38.1	8.1	40.6	7.9	5.3
District of Columbia	100.0	10.3	12.6	63.7	3.1	10.3
Hillsborough County	74.2	37.8	32.6	14.6	5.2	9.8
Los Angeles	97.5	12.9	22.3	62.5	0.0	2.3
Memphis	92.7	31.0	12.0	55.1	0.0	1.9
Miami	81.0	21.3	22.4	35.5	0.0	20.8
Orange County	96.8	9.2	36.9	30.9	3.3	19.8
Philadelphia	92.7	17.8	19.1	53.7	2.3	7.1
San Diego	92.6	37.3	5.9	21.5	5.8	29.5
San Francisco	97.2	6.1	6.5	57.6	0.0	29.8
Local Median	**92.7**	**19.6**	**13.5**	**49.3**	**2.7**	**10.1**
Local Range	**74.2 - 100.0**	**5.8 - 38.1**	**5.9 - 36.9**	**14.6 - 63.7**	**0.0 - 9.1**	**0.0 - 29.8**

* Survey did not include schools from the New York City Department of Education.

TABLE 16. Percentage of All Schools in Which Health Education Staff Worked on Health Education Activities with Other School Staff During the 2005–2006 School Year, Selected U.S. Sites: School Health Profiles, Lead Health Education Teacher Surveys, 2006

Site	Physical education staff	School health services staff	School mental health or social services staff	Nutrition or food service staff
STATE SURVEYS				
Alabama	74.1	78.3	59.8	39.2
Alaska	54.6	42.7	45.9	24.6
Arizona	56.4	47.1	45.9	31.7
Arkansas	79.9	67.7	51.3	37.0
Connecticut	76.5	73.0	65.6	34.1
Delaware	91.1	86.3	74.5	37.8
Florida	56.4	55.2	51.6	30.3
Georgia	90.9	64.4	51.4	33.2
Hawaii	79.9	34.9	38.3	13.5
Idaho	82.2	59.1	63.7	37.2
Iowa	63.8	70.0	44.7	39.0
Kansas	73.9	65.0	43.4	46.2
Maine	78.6	78.7	66.7	43.9
Massachusetts	78.7	74.2	66.7	43.7
Michigan	66.6	28.2	44.2	31.3
Mississippi	58.9	59.2	53.3	42.9
Missouri	83.8	80.6	59.3	41.2
Montana	85.4	56.8	64.6	39.4
Nebraska	71.8	71.5	51.0	37.1
New Hampshire	74.2	76.0	73.8	49.4
New York*	75.9	64.7	66.2	40.2
North Carolina	87.3	74.0	57.2	37.9
North Dakota	68.8	36.4	52.5	45.6
Oregon	76.8	48.7	59.1	30.6
Pennsylvania	89.4	81.0	53.7	42.6
Rhode Island	87.5	72.9	63.7	26.5
South Carolina	76.4	64.0	46.5	31.2
South Dakota	61.5	48.5	40.1	40.1
Tennessee	75.1	69.4	57.3	39.1
Texas	71.8	63.5	40.8	28.4
Utah	76.9	41.0	54.9	20.0
Vermont	77.1	87.8	82.4	48.1
Virginia	88.7	77.2	56.7	31.7
West Virginia	79.3	80.0	67.3	40.2
State Median	**76.7**	**66.4**	**55.8**	**37.9**
State Range	**54.6 - 91.1**	**28.2 - 87.8**	**38.3 - 82.4**	**13.5 - 49.4**

TABLE 16. Percentage of All Schools in Which Health Education Staff Worked on Health Education Activities with Other School Staff During the 2005–2006 School Year, Selected U.S. Sites: School Health Profiles, Lead Health Education Teacher Surveys, 2006 *(continued)*

Site	Physical education staff	School health services staff	School mental health or social services staff	Nutrition or food service staff
LOCAL SURVEYS				
Charlotte-Mecklenburg County	95.1	67.4	59.9	27.3
Chicago	61.3	55.1	56.3	27.7
Dallas	51.0	62.7	37.3	24.0
District of Columbia	75.5	74.8	60.4	39.9
Hillsborough County	53.5	70.4	22.9	19.0
Los Angeles	45.1	67.8	56.2	30.8
Memphis	96.8	76.0	58.5	54.3
Miami	46.8	27.1	46.9	21.3
Orange County	58.5	26.2	38.6	8.5
Philadelphia	83.8	84.8	50.5	53.5
San Diego	51.5	79.6	87.5	9.1
San Francisco	81.2	53.4	67.9	36.7
Local Median	**59.9**	**67.6**	**56.3**	**27.5**
Local Range	**45.1 - 96.8**	**26.2 - 84.8**	**22.9 - 87.5**	**8.5 - 54.3**

* Survey did not include schools from the New York City Department of Education.

TABLE 17. Percentage of All Schools in Which the Major Emphasis of the Lead Health Education Teacher's Professional Preparation Was in a Specific Discipline, Selected U.S. Sites: School Health Profiles, Lead Health Education Teacher Surveys, 2006

Site	Health and physical education combined	Health education only	Physical education only	Other education degree	Kinesiology, exercise science or exercise physiology, home economics or family and consumer science, biology, or other science	Nursing or counseling	Public health, nutrition, or another discipline
STATE SURVEYS*							
Alabama	53.2	10.4	18.7	2.0	11.1	3.8	0.9
Alaska	9.5	4.3	5.8	33.7	21.9	10.3	14.4
Arizona	18.6	2.3	18.9	16.7	14.4	15.1	14.1
Arkansas	67.5	4.6	16.2	1.7	5.7	1.2	3.0
Connecticut	44.1	16.0	18.4	5.2	7.9	3.6	4.8
Delaware	74.2	4.7	12.0	0.0	4.5	1.6	3.0
Florida	26.6	14.2	12.0	14.2	19.7	4.1	9.1
Georgia	78.7	4.0	6.2	2.9	4.3	2.0	2.0
Hawaii	45.6	4.7	16.5	10.3	15.8	0.0	7.1
Idaho	57.5	8.1	12.8	8.7	7.6	1.7	3.7
Iowa	37.3	3.3	13.0	6.5	28.6	4.6	6.8
Kansas	50.8	2.3	26.6	6.3	4.5	7.6	2.0
Maine	40.3	14.9	8.2	10.6	15.3	7.3	3.6
Massachusetts	40.9	21.4	11.4	5.4	6.6	10.6	3.6
Michigan	39.5	9.6	15.3	7.8	23.7	1.7	2.5
Mississippi	47.3	9.7	7.5	2.8	27.1	2.1	3.5
Missouri	56.3	4.1	15.0	3.5	16.4	3.7	1.0
Montana	64.2	1.2	10.5	18.6	3.6	0.6	1.3
Nebraska	38.9	2.3	22.6	2.8	26.9	4.4	2.1
New Hampshire	20.4	21.0	19.7	4.7	12.6	18.2	3.4
New York†	40.8	42.9	6.5	0.7	6.8	1.1	1.2
North Carolina	60.2	3.4	23.3	4.3	5.1	2.6	1.1
North Dakota	40.2	1.7	11.6	12.8	26.3	2.3	5.0
Oregon	45.0	14.3	9.0	12.5	12.0	0.0	7.2
Pennsylvania	88.9	3.0	2.0	3.6	1.2	1.0	0.4
Rhode Island	74.9	7.5	5.0	0.0	0.0	11.2	1.3
South Carolina	45.4	4.2	36.4	3.0	5.7	2.5	2.7
South Dakota	46.2	1.5	6.5	20.3	17.9	2.7	4.8
Tennessee	61.1	3.0	9.5	8.6	6.3	10.1	1.5
Texas	45.2	8.6	9.1	3.8	26.1	3.9	3.3
Utah	45.4	16.0	20.6	5.2	10.3	0.0	2.5
Vermont	36.4	12.9	7.2	5.4	20.8	17.3	0.0
Virginia	81.9	2.4	9.3	3.1	1.9	0.7	0.7
West Virginia	79.2	6.6	6.7	4.7	0.6	0.5	1.8
State Median	**45.5**	**4.7**	**11.8**	**5.2**	**10.7**	**2.7**	**2.9**
State Range	**9.5 – 88.9**	**1.2 – 42.9**	**2.0 – 36.4**	**0.0 – 33.7**	**0.0 – 28.6**	**0.0 – 18.2**	**0.0 – 14.4**

TABLE 17. Percentage of All Schools in Which the Major Emphasis of the Lead Health Education Teacher's Professional Preparation Was in a Specific Discipline, Selected U.S. Sites: School Health Profiles, Lead Health Education Teacher Surveys, 2006 *(continued)*

Site	Health and physical education combined	Health education only	Physical education only	Other education degree	Kinesiology, exercise science or exercise physiology, home economics or family and consumer science, biology, or other science	Nursing or counseling	Public health, nutrition, or another discipline
LOCAL SURVEYS*							
Charlotte-Mecklenburg County	69.7	5.4	22.0	0.0	2.9	0.0	0.0
Chicago	28.2	1.7	24.5	14.0	10.6	15.0	5.6
Dallas	22.4	16.3	0.0	6.1	55.1	0.0	0.0
District of Columbia	82.4	0.0	0.0	0.0	3.4	10.7	3.4
Hillsborough County	32.3	10.6	14.6	10.8	11.4	1.8	18.4
Los Angeles	12.3	29.3	4.7	7.8	32.5	1.2	11.3
Memphis	75.7	4.8	12.5	1.6	5.3	0.0	0.0
Miami	14.5	22.4	22.3	1.4	26.4	9.2	3.9
Orange County	24.6	37.1	14.8	3.0	17.5	0.0	3.0
Philadelphia	85.0	2.3	3.5	2.3	2.3	3.5	1.2
San Diego	1.8	0.0	1.8	10.9	0.0	85.4	0.0
San Francisco	10.0	16.7	3.3	26.7	26.7	6.7	10.0
Local Median	**26.4**	**8.0**	**8.6**	**4.6**	**11.0**	**2.7**	**3.2**
Local Range	**1.8 – 85.0**	**0.0 – 37.1**	**0.0 – 24.5**	**0.0 – 26.7**	**0.0 – 55.1**	**0.0 – 85.4**	**0.0 – 18.4**

* Percentages for each row might not add up to 100.0 because of rounding.

† Survey did not include schools from the New York City Department of Education.

TABLE 18. Percentage of All Schools in Which a Newly Hired Health Education Teacher Was Required to Be Certified* in Health Education, the Lead Health Education Teacher Was Certified in Health Education, or the Lead Health Education Teacher Had Experience Teaching Health Education Classes or Topics for a Specific Number of Years, Selected U.S. Sites: School Health Profiles, Principal Surveys and Lead Health Education Teacher Surveys, 2006

Site	Newly hired health education teacher required to be certified in health education	Lead health education teacher certified in health education	Number of years lead health education teacher taught health education classes or topics				
			1 year	2–5 years	6–9 years	10–14 years	≥15 years
STATE SURVEYS							
Alabama	79.0	78.2	10.3	24.3	17.4	13.6	34.4
Alaska	23.8	26.7	23.1	30.3	19.0	11.4	16.2
Arizona	36.2	31.0	21.3	30.4	13.9	11.8	22.6
Arkansas	94.7	93.7	8.8	26.9	12.3	13.3	38.7
Connecticut	84.3	80.6	5.7	22.3	21.4	12.8	37.8
Delaware	93.9	85.5	7.4	22.3	23.8	22.5	24.0
Florida	65.3	51.1	12.8	23.4	16.1	12.1	35.6
Georgia	88.1	97.2	3.9	19.6	18.6	11.6	46.3
Hawaii	64.1	63.1	6.9	38.4	12.1	20.1	22.5
Idaho	92.9	91.2	5.3	20.2	15.8	21.0	37.7
Illinois	87.6	NA†	NA	NA	NA	NA	NA
Iowa	79.0	75.4	10.7	22.3	15.1	14.8	37.1
Kansas	76.8	71.2	8.6	23.3	17.0	9.7	41.4
Maine	80.1	74.2	9.9	26.5	13.1	10.5	40.1
Massachusetts	84.6	76.9	6.6	20.8	15.7	17.0	39.9
Michigan	90.0	82.2	10.4	28.0	20.8	14.5	26.2
Mississippi	92.1	91.9	8.2	23.2	20.8	14.0	33.7
Missouri	85.1	83.2	8.3	28.9	22.5	15.6	24.6
Montana	85.4	90.8	6.1	20.2	17.5	18.3	37.9
Nebraska	56.7	65.7	8.2	19.4	18.8	15.6	38.0
New Hampshire	68.9	54.2	3.7	25.6	23.8	16.2	30.7
New York‡	97.4	94.6	3.1	22.6	18.8	13.1	42.4
North Carolina	80.2	79.1	6.4	20.9	14.1	14.5	44.0
North Dakota	88.9	93.1	5.3	16.2	16.3	19.6	42.6
Oregon	77.7	78.1	7.2	24.0	14.0	13.5	41.3
Pennsylvania	89.9	95.3	1.7	18.7	14.4	14.3	50.9
Rhode Island	92.8	97.7	3.5	18.9	19.8	19.5	38.3
South Carolina	69.9	74.9	8.5	23.1	16.4	11.0	41.0
South Dakota	81.5	75.5	7.6	30.6	13.0	11.9	36.9
Tennessee	80.1	80.1	7.8	22.5	16.7	14.8	38.2
Texas	87.6	77.7	14.5	24.9	16.8	10.2	33.6
Utah	95.7	89.0	6.9	25.4	19.1	13.4	35.1
Vermont	75.0	62.7	10.2	19.8	14.6	17.8	37.6
Virginia	90.8	93.3	2.9	12.4	13.9	11.4	59.4
Washington	69.2	NA	NA	NA	NA	NA	NA
West Virginia	99.0	94.3	5.2	13.2	13.0	11.3	57.2
State Median	**84.5**	**79.6**	**7.5**	**22.9**	**16.6**	**13.8**	**37.9**
State Range	**23.8 - 99.0**	**26.7 - 97.7**	**1.7 - 23.1**	**12.4 - 38.4**	**12.1 - 23.8**	**9.7 - 22.5**	**16.2 - 59.4**

TABLE 18. Percentage of All Schools in Which a Newly Hired Health Education Teacher Was Required to Be Certified* in Health Education, the Lead Health Education Teacher Was Certified in Health Education, or the Lead Health Education Teacher Had Experience Teaching Health Education Classes or Topics for a Specific Number of Years, Selected U.S. Sites: School Health Profiles, Principal Surveys and Lead Health Education Teacher Surveys, 2006 *(continued)*

Site	Newly hired health education teacher required to be certified in health education	Lead health education teacher certified in health education	Number of years lead health education teacher taught health education classes or topics				
			1 year	2–5 years	6–9 years	10–14 years	≥15 years
LOCAL SURVEYS							
Charlotte-Mecklenburg County	100.0	74.4	2.4	20.2	15.0	27.5	34.8
Chicago	44.3	48.5	10.9	25.2	9.9	14.5	39.5
Dallas	82.6	65.4	12.2	14.3	16.3	12.2	44.9
District of Columbia	93.2	87.4	3.4	19.0	15.9	3.4	58.4
Hillsborough County	76.0	48.4	12.4	21.3	27.5	13.4	25.4
Los Angeles	91.7	77.3	3.6	24.7	32.7	11.1	27.9
Memphis	96.4	84.9	4.7	23.2	14.3	20.7	37.2
Miami	73.4	54.1	12.9	22.1	18.1	14.4	32.4
Orange County	54.2	73.3	8.9	28.8	5.9	17.8	38.6
Philadelphia	75.3	91.7	3.1	12.6	6.1	15.1	63.1
San Diego	0.0	57.8	22.3	48.5	1.9	0.0	27.4
San Francisco	52.2	35.3	29.4	35.3	17.7	8.8	8.8
Local Median	**75.7**	**69.4**	**9.9**	**22.7**	**15.5**	**13.9**	**36.0**
Local Range	**0.0 - 100.0**	**35.3 - 91.7**	**2.4 - 29.4**	**12.6 - 48.5**	**1.9 - 32.7**	**0.0 - 27.5**	**8.8 - 63.1**

* Certification, licensure, or endorsement by the state.
† Data not available.
‡ Survey did not include schools from the New York City Department of Education.

TABLE 19a. Percentage of All Schools in Which the Lead Health Education Teacher Received Staff Development During the 2 Years Preceding the Survey on Specific Health Topics, Selected U.S. Sites: School Health Profiles, Lead Health Education Teacher Surveys, 2006

Site	Alcohol-use or other drug-use prevention	Asthma awareness	Consumer health	CPR*	Dental and oral health	Emotional and mental health	Environmental health
STATE SURVEYS							
Alabama	56.0	30.8	27.5	85.4	14.6	36.9	21.4
Alaska	47.9	14.9	15.4	40.9	13.5	33.1	15.5
Arizona	46.6	24.9	21.4	61.1	19.5	32.8	19.5
Arkansas	52.3	21.5	27.8	70.7	16.8	37.0	16.6
Connecticut	36.3	15.4	16.2	55.0	6.8	34.4	14.1
Delaware	55.9	12.0	18.1	66.8	4.5	34.9	7.7
Florida	51.5	22.1	24.7	63.4	15.5	38.5	18.8
Georgia	49.8	24.3	21.9	72.8	15.1	32.8	15.3
Hawaii	61.8	17.9	42.2	29.6	13.7	47.5	16.0
Idaho	64.6	15.5	35.8	70.1	12.1	48.5	20.5
Iowa	36.3	11.0	17.6	51.2	6.9	25.3	10.9
Kansas	40.7	16.0	20.2	63.7	11.8	27.9	13.2
Maine	41.5	16.6	22.6	53.5	12.7	41.3	14.2
Massachusetts	47.6	15.1	15.6	63.7	11.0	41.6	11.4
Michigan	40.8	24.9	18.0	55.2	6.6	30.1	11.3
Mississippi	61.2	25.1	40.9	60.9	22.7	39.3	20.5
Missouri	49.3	26.2	22.3	68.8	13.8	32.1	11.9
Montana	70.0	13.8	24.1	71.4	9.5	38.9	13.4
Nebraska	49.1	57.4	16.2	65.3	7.7	27.1	9.8
New Hampshire	68.1	17.4	35.8	68.2	13.2	62.3	19.9
New York†	55.2	13.0	24.0	73.0	6.2	47.0	15.1
North Carolina	42.5	30.6	18.9	67.7	9.6	25.6	12.7
North Dakota	57.7	17.6	27.8	59.3	10.2	36.3	13.5
Oregon	56.1	21.1	17.9	74.8	13.5	38.0	15.9
Pennsylvania	52.3	23.6	19.8	78.6	7.4	40.0	10.2
Rhode Island	37.7	14.8	14.0	67.1	3.5	26.6	9.3
South Carolina	37.5	17.5	22.8	66.5	14.4	25.3	16.0
South Dakota	45.3	17.8	20.1	69.4	11.4	23.8	9.6
Tennessee	53.6	28.6	26.8	69.0	20.1	41.2	18.5
Texas	46.6	21.7	23.8	82.6	13.6	27.4	17.4
Utah	63.0	19.0	23.1	68.2	7.8	43.4	7.8
Vermont	67.2	22.5	19.2	53.5	12.5	42.6	13.3
Virginia	47.8	24.0	23.4	78.0	8.4	31.9	13.5
West Virginia	50.9	19.4	22.0	55.0	14.7	28.8	15.2
State Median	**50.4**	**19.2**	**22.2**	**67.0**	**12.3**	**35.6**	**14.2**
State Range	**36.3 - 70.0**	**11.0 - 57.4**	**14.0 - 42.2**	**29.6 - 85.4**	**3.5 - 22.7**	**23.8 - 62.3**	**7.7 - 21.4**

TABLE 19a. Percentage of All Schools in Which the Lead Health Education Teacher Received Staff Development During the 2 Years Preceding the Survey on Specific Health Topics, Selected U.S. Sites: School Health Profiles, Lead Health Education Teacher Surveys, 2006 *(continued)*

Site	Alcohol-use or other drug-use prevention	Asthma awareness	Consumer health	CPR*	Dental and oral health	Emotional and mental health	Environmental health
LOCAL SURVEYS							
Charlotte-Mecklenburg County	67.2	54.9	43.7	77.1	15.0	50.4	22.9
Chicago	39.1	48.0	25.8	40.6	29.8	35.5	24.3
Dallas	66.0	13.7	28.0	62.7	13.5	33.3	24.0
District of Columbia	44.5	34.9	35.5	38.2	29.3	48.6	38.9
Hillsborough County	39.0	32.7	17.2	76.6	5.0	18.4	14.5
Los Angeles	78.2	35.1	24.7	48.1	15.1	48.1	29.1
Memphis	71.7	67.4	53.3	88.0	37.3	54.5	38.5
Miami	42.0	11.3	29.7	59.7	13.8	27.7	17.8
Orange County	62.9	5.9	17.4	56.4	14.2	42.4	14.5
Philadelphia	41.7	68.0	19.4	87.9	14.6	32.8	11.8
San Diego	100.0	11.2	40.9	43.0	5.4	86.7	7.5
San Francisco	87.9	21.2	27.3	39.4	12.5	56.2	9.1
Local Median	**64.5**	**33.8**	**27.7**	**58.1**	**14.4**	**45.3**	**20.4**
Local Range	**39.0 - 100.0**	**5.9 - 68.0**	**17.2 - 53.3**	**38.2 - 88.0**	**5.0 - 37.3**	**18.4 - 86.7**	**7.5 - 38.9**

* Cardiopulmonary resuscitation.
† Survey did not include schools from the New York City Department of Education.

TABLE 19b. Percentage of All Schools in Which the Lead Health Education Teacher Received Staff Development During the 2 Years Preceding the Survey on Specific Health Topics, Selected U.S. Sites: School Health Profiles, Lead Health Education Teacher Surveys, 2006

Site	First aid	Foodborne illness prevention	Growth and development	HIV* prevention	Human sexuality	Immunizations	Injury prevention and safety
STATE SURVEYS							
Alabama	77.1	24.3	25.8	54.7	32.3	21.3	58.6
Alaska	46.6	20.1	20.7	25.7	15.5	22.8	30.5
Arizona	55.5	22.1	27.5	32.4	19.3	30.7	43.0
Arkansas	66.8	15.3	21.9	30.6	19.8	16.9	52.5
Connecticut	50.7	13.6	23.4	39.0	29.5	10.8	34.3
Delaware	48.6	9.2	24.2	39.5	39.6	13.6	25.9
Florida	59.4	18.9	31.4	56.3	36.9	21.5	43.7
Georgia	60.4	15.1	31.9	50.0	38.4	15.6	42.6
Hawaii	29.1	19.5	25.6	53.4	46.2	7.4	36.8
Idaho	65.8	16.3	21.3	48.3	35.9	15.2	44.4
Iowa	41.6	21.1	17.9	32.6	18.1	20.9	26.3
Kansas	55.3	19.5	25.1	43.9	42.0	16.9	33.0
Maine	45.7	15.4	29.1	43.4	35.9	11.7	36.1
Massachusetts	45.8	13.6	26.1	28.9	29.5	12.0	33.4
Michigan	47.5	17.0	29.8	57.2	48.9	8.2	29.2
Mississippi	52.8	25.6	27.1	41.0	30.9	24.7	48.2
Missouri	66.0	21.9	27.9	34.3	23.3	18.4	49.9
Montana	72.2	21.3	23.6	44.8	27.1	13.5	47.9
Nebraska	50.6	17.4	20.8	29.5	24.6	18.2	29.2
New Hampshire	57.9	21.1	49.8	63.9	65.6	13.2	43.9
New York†	61.2	13.1	28.2	52.5	39.0	10.9	38.3
North Carolina	64.2	18.9	24.1	48.2	37.1	12.9	44.8
North Dakota	48.3	30.2	22.6	32.5	20.4	21.1	31.3
Oregon	75.1	21.8	22.7	48.7	39.9	12.2	41.8
Pennsylvania	59.1	9.2	20.7	37.8	26.6	9.2	41.4
Rhode Island	53.5	20.9	19.4	24.3	12.7	16.2	36.7
South Carolina	64.2	19.1	30.8	51.3	41.9	18.1	42.3
South Dakota	47.5	14.3	18.1	21.3	15.8	17.0	25.0
Tennessee	66.0	19.3	26.6	51.0	25.1	22.8	52.7
Texas	71.7	18.3	25.9	35.0	29.9	20.5	52.5
Utah	61.4	14.9	29.5	53.6	60.5	11.4	35.9
Vermont	41.6	19.3	33.3	44.2	40.6	18.0	28.3
Virginia	64.9	16.5	30.8	45.0	41.2	18.1	44.4
West Virginia	46.5	14.8	22.4	24.0	18.9	12.5	30.2
State Median	**56.7**	**18.9**	**25.7**	**43.7**	**31.6**	**16.6**	**39.9**
State Range	**29.1 - 77.1**	**9.2 - 30.2**	**17.9 - 49.8**	**21.3 - 63.9**	**12.7 - 65.6**	**7.4 - 30.7**	**25.0 - 58.6**

TABLE 19b. Percentage of All Schools in Which the Lead Health Education Teacher Received Staff Development During the 2 Years Preceding the Survey on Specific Health Topics, Selected U.S. Sites: School Health Profiles, Lead Health Education Teacher Surveys, 2006 *(continued)*

Site	First aid	Foodborne illness prevention	Growth and development	HIV* prevention	Human sexuality	Immunizations	Injury prevention and safety
LOCAL SURVEYS							
Charlotte-Mecklenburg County	79.8	20.0	57.3	62.4	79.6	17.6	67.4
Chicago	44.0	21.2	35.6	42.9	33.4	33.9	41.3
Dallas	51.9	26.0	65.4	61.5	65.4	19.6	53.8
District of Columbia	47.2	23.7	48.9	65.9	50.3	29.3	38.9
Hillsborough County	63.1	14.6	26.3	58.9	32.2	16.9	34.4
Los Angeles	41.7	22.1	37.6	82.5	62.1	25.6	43.3
Memphis	90.0	38.5	54.0	89.2	71.0	36.9	75.8
Miami	49.5	17.6	49.5	69.2	43.2	22.5	37.6
Orange County	53.4	14.2	45.4	88.1	76.6	22.8	42.4
Philadelphia	71.3	13.6	34.5	52.4	44.1	14.0	50.4
San Diego	24.3	14.6	63.0	100.0	100.0	36.6	24.5
San Francisco	36.3	6.1	21.2	60.6	66.7	6.1	34.4
Local Median	**50.7**	**18.8**	**47.2**	**64.2**	**63.8**	**22.7**	**41.9**
Local Range	**24.3 - 90.0**	**6.1 - 38.5**	**21.2 - 65.4**	**42.9 - 100.0**	**32.2 - 100.0**	**6.1 - 36.9**	**24.5 - 75.8**

* Human immunodeficiency virus.

† Survey did not include schools from the New York City Department of Education.

TABLE 19c. Percentage of All Schools in Which the Lead Health Education Teacher Received Staff Development During the 2 Years Preceding the Survey on Specific Health Topics, Selected U.S. Sites: School Health Profiles, Lead Health Education Teacher Surveys, 2006

Site	Nutrition and dietary behavior	Physical activity and fitness	Pregnancy prevention	STD* prevention	Suicide prevention	Sun safety or skin cancer prevention	Tobacco-use prevention	Violence prevention
STATE SURVEYS								
Alabama	35.4	52.4	34.4	44.0	24.0	17.4	35.1	59.7
Alaska	21.3	29.9	12.6	21.5	34.5	6.8	26.0	50.8
Arizona	30.5	39.6	16.3	23.2	25.9	26.8	37.9	59.4
Arkansas	39.9	56.7	22.7	26.0	28.3	14.2	49.0	60.9
Connecticut	35.1	44.0	22.8	32.2	20.4	8.9	21.1	45.9
Delaware	27.4	51.7	36.5	39.6	15.3	7.6	40.7	51.5
Florida	46.0	48.1	34.9	46.3	31.6	26.9	36.1	57.0
Georgia	30.4	49.7	39.6	48.4	25.7	14.1	34.2	45.4
Hawaii	52.6	58.9	46.0	47.1	25.2	15.6	46.8	56.3
Idaho	46.9	48.1	26.9	42.6	39.6	16.0	41.6	54.0
Iowa	30.3	27.5	15.0	23.0	15.5	8.5	16.7	46.7
Kansas	39.1	54.2	29.8	39.4	20.6	10.5	26.3	50.1
Maine	40.9	45.7	30.1	36.7	39.1	20.9	32.9	49.0
Massachusetts	43.9	45.1	22.0	26.8	28.4	43.1	25.7	61.2
Michigan	35.3	42.6	37.0	50.3	20.5	9.1	26.4	47.7
Mississippi	47.4	42.6	33.4	37.4	27.3	19.6	46.4	45.5
Missouri	40.2	53.2	21.3	30.8	24.6	14.2	32.0	52.9
Montana	34.5	51.9	23.4	33.2	30.7	10.3	39.4	58.6
Nebraska	30.3	37.7	23.0	28.8	22.4	11.0	27.7	51.6
New Hampshire	72.8	64.6	55.7	64.8	25.8	21.1	45.0	49.8
New York†	44.9	41.4	32.1	41.9	27.0	13.1	38.9	64.5
North Carolina	33.0	58.4	35.6	43.9	17.9	17.3	37.7	51.5
North Dakota	40.8	44.9	13.6	29.6	33.9	12.0	42.4	57.6
Oregon	27.5	35.2	35.0	45.7	30.3	10.0	35.0	57.5
Pennsylvania	43.5	58.0	21.2	30.7	22.1	8.4	31.5	56.3
Rhode Island	27.5	39.8	10.3	17.4	14.8	8.1	19.4	45.1
South Carolina	27.5	56.8	36.3	41.6	11.4	12.2	26.2	41.5
South Dakota	34.6	34.4	11.3	18.0	21.7	9.4	25.6	40.7
Tennessee	34.8	51.0	24.5	35.9	31.4	14.3	31.4	62.8
Texas	28.8	48.4	25.7	31.8	21.0	18.2	30.2	49.0
Utah	38.1	51.7	35.2	47.6	30.0	15.8	49.7	47.6
Vermont	46.4	45.6	28.0	37.9	24.2	11.6	43.0	70.1
Virginia	36.1	64.4	28.8	36.6	38.5	13.1	30.8	67.2
West Virginia	29.4	60.4	22.4	22.8	14.2	13.7	49.0	54.0
State Median	**35.4**	**48.3**	**27.5**	**36.7**	**25.5**	**13.4**	**34.6**	**52.3**
State Range	**21.3 – 72.8**	**27.5 – 64.6**	**10.3 – 55.7**	**17.4 – 64.8**	**11.4 – 39.6**	**6.8 – 43.1**	**16.7 – 49.7**	**40.7 – 70.1**

TABLE 19c. Percentage of All Schools in Which the Lead Health Education Teacher Received Staff Development During the 2 Years Preceding the Survey on Specific Health Topics, Selected U.S. Sites: School Health Profiles, Lead Health Education Teacher Surveys, 2006 *(continued)*

Site	Nutrition and dietary behavior	Physical activity and fitness	Pregnancy prevention	STD* prevention	Suicide prevention	Sun safety or skin cancer prevention	Tobacco-use prevention	Violence prevention
LOCAL SURVEYS								
Charlotte-Mecklenburg County	50.4	77.3	62.5	60.1	39.0	46.1	37.6	77.3
Chicago	38.6	54.2	30.4	35.4	21.3	11.8	34.7	58.7
Dallas	41.2	32.7	42.0	61.5	28.8	19.6	50.0	61.5
District of Columbia	45.5	48.6	39.2	56.9	29.3	22.4	41.2	55.1
Hillsborough County	32.4	47.7	22.9	37.6	16.3	12.6	28.1	55.0
Los Angeles	40.8	34.6	53.8	70.8	32.6	17.2	85.5	69.9
Memphis	51.1	81.2	64.0	89.1	42.9	29.8	51.1	76.6
Miami	35.1	46.1	43.2	57.3	25.0	26.3	29.8	44.0
Orange County	48.1	40.1	65.6	79.8	36.5	23.1	40.1	60.2
Philadelphia	63.2	80.3	27.2	42.0	20.3	11.7	35.8	68.0
San Diego	21.8	23.6	92.8	100.0	82.8	10.7	100.0	81.4
San Francisco	63.6	39.4	41.9	54.6	34.4	6.1	87.9	72.7
Local Median	**43.4**	**46.9**	**42.6**	**58.7**	**31.0**	**18.4**	**40.7**	**64.8**
Local Range	**21.8 - 63.6**	**23.6 - 81.2**	**22.9 - 92.8**	**35.4 - 100.0**	**16.3 - 82.8**	**6.1 - 46.1**	**28.1 - 100.0**	**44.0 - 81.4**

* Sexually transmitted disease.
† Survey did not include schools from the New York City Department of Education.

TABLE 20a. Percentage of All Schools in Which the Lead Health Education Teacher Wanted to Receive Staff Development on Specific Health Topics, Selected U.S. Sites: School Health Profiles, Lead Health Education Teacher Surveys, 2006

Site	Alcohol-use or other drug-use prevention	Asthma awareness	Consumer health	CPR*	Dental and oral health	Emotional and mental health	Environmental health	First aid
STATE SURVEYS								
Alabama	76.5	68.3	53.5	68.4	55.1	70.6	50.3	67.6
Alaska	67.8	54.1	48.6	64.9	45.3	71.6	52.7	64.9
Arizona	70.5	60.3	48.5	66.9	42.8	64.8	52.3	67.4
Arkansas	79.7	61.7	54.9	71.4	49.8	66.4	52.4	79.6
Connecticut	73.3	56.6	62.2	55.9	41.7	78.7	55.7	56.3
Delaware	78.4	54.3	44.6	59.5	35.6	71.4	44.5	67.0
Florida	74.3	59.5	57.0	70.1	49.9	71.9	55.4	70.1
Georgia	79.2	63.6	50.1	71.1	49.0	67.3	55.7	76.0
Hawaii	69.3	58.9	64.6	69.0	53.9	64.5	61.5	67.8
Idaho	73.1	53.8	47.6	65.3	43.4	69.7	52.5	66.6
Iowa	60.5	44.2	41.9	60.4	28.6	62.2	42.5	57.0
Kansas	70.3	50.4	42.9	63.9	34.6	62.6	39.5	60.7
Maine	60.9	42.9	47.1	53.8	32.1	63.7	42.8	59.1
Massachusetts	78.8	55.8	59.3	65.2	43.8	78.8	57.4	67.7
Michigan	67.8	53.6	51.2	62.5	39.1	67.4	48.1	63.8
Mississippi	79.7	64.4	58.8	78.4	57.4	71.7	58.6	78.8
Missouri	68.8	51.3	48.0	67.1	42.0	65.5	45.3	67.8
Montana	71.8	61.2	44.7	61.0	43.4	70.7	46.9	63.2
Nebraska	61.5	43.5	36.1	55.3	33.7	55.6	37.7	54.6
New Hampshire	76.4	56.6	62.3	51.8	46.4	78.5	65.9	54.5
New York†	81.4	54.1	62.8	60.4	41.7	79.4	59.8	60.1
North Carolina	70.0	64.4	47.2	69.5	42.2	62.3	45.5	72.8
North Dakota	55.9	51.8	44.2	63.5	30.4	63.3	37.1	61.4
Oregon	65.0	44.7	44.7	48.9	38.5	67.4	54.2	52.0
Pennsylvania	78.2	61.7	62.4	68.6	46.0	76.1	58.1	71.0
Rhode Island	74.6	56.4	65.5	54.0	35.0	76.6	57.6	56.5
South Carolina	70.5	57.6	45.7	67.2	45.3	64.8	48.4	61.3
South Dakota	54.7	47.9	48.3	61.4	34.4	57.7	37.2	63.8
Tennessee	76.5	61.2	54.4	72.2	50.4	72.1	54.1	76.1
Texas	74.0	57.3	51.0	67.2	46.9	69.4	55.6	69.1
Utah	73.5	51.0	55.6	63.2	39.6	80.2	53.3	65.2
Vermont	53.7	33.0	46.3	49.0	27.0	61.4	42.0	50.2
Virginia	63.1	62.3	44.3	61.1	37.4	61.0	43.6	59.9
West Virginia	73.4	65.9	53.0	74.3	45.7	63.3	56.2	76.7
State Median	**72.5**	**56.5**	**49.4**	**64.4**	**42.5**	**67.4**	**52.5**	**65.1**
State Range	**53.7 – 81.4**	**33.0 – 68.3**	**36.1 – 65.5**	**48.9 – 78.4**	**27.0 – 57.4**	**55.6 – 80.2**	**37.1 – 65.9**	**50.2 – 79.6**

TABLE 20a. Percentage of All Schools in Which the Lead Health Education Teacher Wanted to Receive Staff Development on Specific Health Topics, Selected U.S. Sites: School Health Profiles, Lead Health Education Teacher Surveys, 2006 *(continued)*

Site	Alcohol-use or other drug-use prevention	Asthma awareness	Consumer health	CPR*	Dental and oral health	Emotional and mental health	Environmental health	First aid
LOCAL SURVEYS								
Charlotte-Mecklenburg County	74.5	72.0	61.8	74.5	51.1	77.4	61.6	67.0
Chicago	67.9	71.4	59.7	83.5	57.0	77.9	56.7	82.9
Dallas	80.4	66.7	56.3	75.0	51.0	76.9	62.7	79.6
District of Columbia	81.2	84.1	74.1	84.1	70.7	83.5	80.6	84.4
Hillsborough County	48.3	35.3	35.2	66.4	33.6	62.9	39.4	67.8
Los Angeles	73.3	65.6	66.6	70.4	56.1	77.0	68.5	72.8
Memphis	85.9	85.2	74.5	84.6	76.3	82.9	71.1	81.5
Miami	73.1	62.7	57.5	76.5	53.7	73.2	58.5	74.4
Orange County	73.9	46.3	46.0	62.9	48.4	68.5	51.3	63.5
Philadelphia	76.3	80.2	67.0	78.6	62.0	79.5	72.6	76.5
San Diego	81.8	50.1	60.9	60.6	39.1	87.4	38.6	56.8
San Francisco	77.4	46.9	56.3	60.6	45.4	87.5	60.6	71.9
Local Median	**75.4**	**66.2**	**60.3**	**74.8**	**52.4**	**77.7**	**61.1**	**73.6**
Local Range	**48.3 - 85.9**	**35.3 - 85.2**	**35.2 - 74.5**	**60.6 - 84.6**	**33.6 - 76.3**	**62.9 - 87.5**	**38.6 - 80.6**	**56.8 - 84.4**

* Cardiopulmonary resuscitation.
† Survey did not include schools from the New York City Department of Education.

TABLE 20b. Percentage of All Schools in Which the Lead Health Education Teacher Wanted to Receive Staff Development on Specific Health Topics, Selected U.S. Sites: School Health Profiles, Lead Health Education Teacher Surveys, 2006

Site	Foodborne illness prevention	Growth and development	HIV* prevention	Human sexuality	Immunizations	Injury prevention and safety	Nutrition and dietary behavior
STATE SURVEYS							
Alabama	53.4	56.8	68.3	59.4	53.1	69.1	74.8
Alaska	48.1	55.4	57.3	53.5	44.5	58.0	66.0
Arizona	45.0	51.8	55.9	48.2	42.1	61.9	64.7
Arkansas	55.7	59.1	66.2	56.9	47.3	72.4	75.9
Connecticut	54.6	64.6	69.7	68.4	45.6	55.1	76.7
Delaware	44.7	59.6	66.3	71.4	41.6	56.6	72.6
Florida	59.8	61.4	69.3	66.2	53.9	65.2	73.2
Georgia	57.9	60.9	70.9	61.5	46.4	70.6	74.4
Hawaii	61.4	57.3	54.6	55.1	59.5	53.0	68.3
Idaho	49.7	54.8	64.3	59.2	47.4	58.5	74.9
Iowa	38.5	45.9	55.0	50.3	38.2	47.7	62.2
Kansas	40.4	55.9	60.0	58.3	40.8	53.3	71.7
Maine	37.0	43.7	46.1	46.3	31.4	50.0	62.2
Massachusetts	53.3	63.1	70.7	75.0	45.9	62.5	76.5
Michigan	47.0	50.0	57.6	57.6	43.3	57.3	67.3
Mississippi	61.0	59.3	74.9	60.3	57.5	70.7	68.0
Missouri	44.7	52.8	63.4	55.1	44.1	62.3	69.2
Montana	49.8	56.6	62.4	56.1	50.3	62.4	73.9
Nebraska	35.8	40.7	54.1	49.3	34.9	46.2	57.3
New Hampshire	53.7	60.7	62.1	66.0	50.8	67.3	78.0
New York†	51.1	66.0	74.7	73.0	52.0	55.8	76.1
North Carolina	48.2	52.9	61.7	55.5	43.4	66.3	75.2
North Dakota	42.7	45.0	54.4	53.0	37.3	48.2	60.3
Oregon	42.5	54.1	57.8	56.1	40.4	47.1	67.1
Pennsylvania	56.8	67.0	77.4	75.4	53.0	65.0	78.5
Rhode Island	51.8	55.9	70.2	66.7	44.4	62.0	77.9
South Carolina	46.2	51.6	64.2	55.7	42.7	56.1	74.2
South Dakota	37.1	39.4	48.4	40.9	33.8	51.1	66.4
Tennessee	55.4	59.5	63.5	54.6	48.3	69.5	73.2
Texas	58.3	58.1	65.0	59.6	49.1	63.5	74.0
Utah	50.5	57.4	66.7	66.0	47.1	60.7	78.5
Vermont	36.4	41.5	46.2	47.5	30.7	42.0	64.9
Virginia	45.7	47.3	47.2	45.2	41.1	55.1	72.7
West Virginia	59.4	53.2	64.7	60.0	49.0	65.7	76.6
State Median	**49.8**	**55.9**	**63.5**	**57.3**	**45.1**	**59.6**	**73.2**
State Range	**35.8 - 61.4**	**39.4 - 67.0**	**46.1 - 77.4**	**40.9 - 75.4**	**30.7 - 59.5**	**42.0 - 72.4**	**57.3 - 78.5**

TABLE 20b. Percentage of All Schools in Which the Lead Health Education Teacher Wanted to Receive Staff Development on Specific Health Topics, Selected U.S. Sites: School Health Profiles, Lead Health Education Teacher Surveys, 2006 *(continued)*

Site	Foodborne illness prevention	Growth and development	HIV* prevention	Human sexuality	Immunizations	Injury prevention and safety	Nutrition and dietary behavior
LOCAL SURVEYS							
Charlotte-Mecklenburg County	61.4	64.3	67.0	56.4	51.2	64.1	77.2
Chicago	61.1	65.4	66.9	62.8	57.8	67.9	73.4
Dallas	68.6	65.4	76.0	72.0	60.8	59.2	76.9
District of Columbia	80.6	77.3	83.8	80.6	73.8	77.3	81.2
Hillsborough County	41.9	47.8	60.5	50.5	41.5	48.3	58.6
Los Angeles	68.2	66.8	72.5	72.6	67.8	56.5	71.8
Memphis	72.6	83.8	84.6	79.5	80.3	78.6	83.1
Miami	59.8	61.0	70.7	67.2	53.7	71.5	79.3
Orange County	51.6	47.3	62.6	62.6	33.8	49.0	71.2
Philadelphia	72.7	76.1	78.7	78.3	66.7	75.7	77.0
San Diego	42.5	51.6	69.4	63.9	44.0	42.5	58.5
San Francisco	39.4	56.2	63.6	71.0	48.4	64.5	75.7
Local Median	**61.3**	**64.8**	**70.1**	**69.1**	**55.8**	**64.3**	**76.3**
Local Range	**39.4 - 80.6**	**47.3 - 83.8**	**60.5 - 84.6**	**50.5 - 80.6**	**33.8 - 80.3**	**42.5 - 78.6**	**58.5 - 83.1**

* Human immunodeficiency virus.

† Survey did not include schools from the New York City Department of Education.

TABLE 20c. Percentage of All Schools in Which the Lead Health Education Teacher Wanted to Receive Staff Development on Specific Health Topics, Selected U.S. Sites: School Health Profiles, Lead Health Education Teacher Surveys, 2006

Site	Physical activity and fitness	Pregnancy prevention	STD* prevention	Suicide prevention	Sun safety or skin cancer prevention	Tobacco-use prevention	Violence prevention
STATE SURVEYS							
Alabama	71.1	62.7	71.2	75.5	60.3	70.2	79.6
Alaska	60.3	53.5	55.8	72.3	42.2	63.1	68.2
Arizona	57.6	53.0	54.7	66.1	59.8	60.3	72.5
Arkansas	78.5	59.6	67.4	77.9	58.6	74.3	77.9
Connecticut	62.3	62.6	68.4	77.6	58.0	65.5	76.1
Delaware	68.4	61.9	66.7	69.9	47.5	66.9	83.5
Florida	68.7	65.6	68.0	72.9	66.1	65.6	75.3
Georgia	72.1	62.1	68.3	74.8	60.9	71.5	82.3
Hawaii	58.7	59.2	56.4	72.4	62.8	64.6	81.3
Idaho	69.4	55.9	60.7	74.6	53.0	62.9	79.3
Iowa	60.1	52.0	54.4	69.3	47.9	53.2	67.0
Kansas	68.8	57.3	64.1	68.9	49.7	63.9	70.7
Maine	52.7	44.6	52.6	65.9	44.0	50.3	66.8
Massachusetts	69.7	66.6	74.0	82.4	57.3	64.0	80.9
Michigan	64.8	53.0	57.1	68.8	51.3	57.3	70.7
Mississippi	70.3	71.3	74.4	80.5	65.0	70.8	83.5
Missouri	66.6	58.1	62.5	69.9	49.9	59.4	74.9
Montana	71.5	57.1	61.5	71.7	50.0	59.9	72.1
Nebraska	53.8	49.6	53.3	63.2	40.0	57.3	66.8
New Hampshire	68.6	58.8	68.3	73.9	64.9	64.8	76.7
New York†	69.9	69.2	75.0	85.2	60.3	65.7	83.6
North Carolina	75.4	57.6	62.2	68.8	56.7	64.2	76.4
North Dakota	60.4	42.8	55.8	71.0	46.7	51.9	69.0
Oregon	58.8	51.9	55.8	67.6	50.8	53.5	67.2
Pennsylvania	75.8	72.3	77.7	81.8	60.1	73.3	78.6
Rhode Island	64.4	63.4	63.2	72.3	55.1	51.9	81.4
South Carolina	71.1	57.4	61.9	68.3	50.8	59.9	76.6
South Dakota	60.9	39.5	47.9	62.6	41.7	46.6	65.0
Tennessee	75.0	59.3	63.6	74.5	58.4	67.0	81.3
Texas	65.7	58.3	63.0	76.5	57.8	65.8	77.7
Utah	67.9	54.8	65.2	74.2	57.9	61.0	79.5
Vermont	50.9	46.6	47.9	64.4	42.6	45.1	58.7
Virginia	67.7	46.2	46.2	63.8	53.5	56.2	73.9
West Virginia	67.3	65.3	65.2	75.9	60.9	64.4	74.0
State Median	**67.8**	**57.9**	**62.8**	**72.3**	**55.9**	**63.5**	**76.3**
State Range	**50.9 - 78.5**	**39.5 - 72.3**	**46.2 - 77.7**	**62.6 - 85.2**	**40.0 - 66.1**	**45.1 - 74.3**	**58.7 - 83.6**

TABLE 20c. Percentage of All Schools in Which the Lead Health Education Teacher Wanted to Receive Staff Development on Specific Health Topics, Selected U.S. Sites: School Health Profiles, Lead Health Education Teacher Surveys, 2006 *(continued)*

Site	Physical activity and fitness	Pregnancy prevention	STD* prevention	Suicide prevention	Sun safety or skin cancer prevention	Tobacco-use prevention	Violence prevention
LOCAL SURVEYS							
Charlotte-Mecklenburg County	61.6	56.4	64.3	71.8	61.6	66.6	81.9
Chicago	68.9	62.1	68.1	74.4	57.9	65.9	85.7
Dallas	65.3	68.6	74.0	78.8	52.9	66.0	78.4
District of Columbia	83.8	83.8	83.8	78.6	73.8	83.8	93.7
Hillsborough County	46.8	49.3	55.1	62.9	61.3	52.4	63.4
Los Angeles	65.7	69.0	71.4	82.9	58.6	58.8	83.2
Memphis	81.8	84.4	88.0	86.3	69.0	74.1	83.1
Miami	75.6	63.9	64.7	70.8	64.5	58.5	69.8
Orange County	51.3	65.3	68.5	73.6	49.7	61.6	73.6
Philadelphia	73.6	78.3	75.2	85.9	69.6	71.4	80.2
San Diego	55.0	72.7	72.6	96.3	42.8	68.8	94.8
San Francisco	71.0	65.6	66.7	75.8	43.7	51.5	87.9
Local Median	**67.3**	**67.1**	**70.0**	**77.2**	**60.0**	**66.0**	**82.5**
Local Range	**46.8 - 83.8**	**49.3 - 84.4**	**55.1 - 88.0**	**62.9 - 96.3**	**42.8 - 73.8**	**51.5 - 83.8**	**63.4 - 94.8**

* Sexually transmitted disease.
† Survey did not include schools from the New York City Department of Education.

TABLE 21. Percentage of All Schools in Which the Lead Health Education Teacher Received Staff Development During the 2 Years Preceding the Survey on Specific Topics, Selected U.S. Sites: School Health Profiles, Lead Health Education Teacher Surveys, 2006

Site	Teaching students with physical or cognitive disabilities	Teaching students of various cultural backgrounds	Teaching students with limited English proficiency	Using interactive teaching methods	Encouraging family or community involvement	Teaching skills for behavior change	Classroom management techniques	Assessing or evaluating students in health education
STATE SURVEYS								
Alabama	63.0	46.4	42.5	50.5	50.6	56.0	72.9	30.6
Alaska	55.3	65.9	40.2	50.8	50.3	43.2	50.4	28.2
Arizona	59.1	63.8	77.9	61.3	47.5	51.7	65.1	27.0
Arkansas	54.3	49.5	33.4	56.1	72.0	59.1	75.7	39.6
Connecticut	53.4	33.2	18.6	47.1	26.1	46.2	55.2	49.2
Delaware	46.3	47.8	25.4	50.8	32.8	46.1	59.7	46.4
Florida	52.6	60.6	58.8	66.1	47.1	58.9	70.9	30.1
Georgia	38.8	38.8	28.8	53.4	33.6	39.1	53.1	27.4
Hawaii	36.6	42.4	32.5	54.2	31.0	43.0	53.0	66.7
Idaho	43.3	38.4	39.5	46.3	35.1	41.8	45.8	26.5
Iowa	52.9	43.9	26.3	55.6	38.7	50.5	56.3	21.0
Kansas	39.0	35.9	21.4	49.7	38.0	40.9	48.7	24.9
Maine	39.2	12.5	7.6	46.1	27.5	37.8	39.4	58.3
Massachusetts	50.9	37.8	34.1	44.9	30.1	44.4	54.2	36.7
Michigan	41.2	30.3	17.4	52.2	33.8	43.3	53.5	24.9
Mississippi	52.9	40.4	22.3	56.5	49.3	54.3	73.0	36.6
Missouri	52.0	42.9	21.1	63.1	53.4	56.3	72.8	37.4
Montana	43.6	33.0	8.8	45.2	35.8	52.7	57.2	34.6
Nebraska	35.1	30.6	20.2	40.1	29.1	39.5	50.3	21.4
New Hampshire	64.9	20.6	8.8	68.0	43.1	61.1	63.4	60.7
New York*	52.7	34.5	16.6	56.2	36.5	52.7	56.7	39.6
North Carolina	47.0	47.1	31.3	52.0	35.2	45.7	63.7	32.2
North Dakota	49.5	25.3	13.4	43.5	33.9	43.2	56.6	15.2
Oregon	49.7	54.8	53.8	54.0	37.2	52.2	57.0	33.2
Pennsylvania	54.0	35.3	33.0	46.0	30.7	45.0	58.1	35.3
Rhode Island	37.0	26.9	18.6	44.5	39.4	32.8	47.9	31.2
South Carolina	39.5	44.9	29.1	51.2	42.2	46.1	64.4	30.0
South Dakota	43.4	22.7	9.5	35.7	32.2	31.6	49.3	22.7
Tennessee	48.3	41.8	25.4	59.6	53.6	49.6	66.1	30.3
Texas	58.9	52.1	51.0	54.9	44.5	56.3	70.9	30.7
Utah	43.4	46.9	49.8	55.7	35.0	42.3	53.2	30.2
Vermont	52.2	24.4	13.0	54.8	38.2	54.9	58.2	55.0
Virginia	51.8	42.5	29.3	61.3	38.2	46.2	62.8	31.6
West Virginia	48.4	37.1	11.0	52.0	35.4	48.4	65.9	39.1
State Median	**49.6**	**39.6**	**25.9**	**52.1**	**36.9**	**46.2**	**57.1**	**31.4**
State Range	**35.1 - 64.9**	**12.5 - 65.9**	**7.6 - 77.9**	**35.7 - 68.0**	**26.1 - 72.0**	**31.6 - 61.1**	**39.4 - 75.7**	**15.2 - 66.7**

TABLE 21. Percentage of All Schools in Which the Lead Health Education Teacher Received Staff Development During the 2 Years Preceding the Survey on Specific Topics, Selected U.S. Sites: School Health Profiles, Lead Health Education Teacher Surveys, 2006 *(continued)*

Site	Teaching students with physical or cognitive disabilities	Teaching students of various cultural backgrounds	Teaching students with limited English proficiency	Using interactive teaching methods	Encouraging family or community involvement	Teaching skills for behavior change	Classroom management techniques	Assessing or evaluating students in health education
LOCAL SURVEYS								
Charlotte-Mecklenburg County	57.2	69.3	48.9	89.8	61.6	61.4	74.5	82.2
Chicago	66.2	50.7	39.3	67.6	54.9	62.6	67.8	29.0
Dallas	57.7	59.6	50.0	73.1	51.9	61.5	90.2	34.6
District of Columbia	40.7	21.7	18.7	59.6	37.4	48.4	49.7	40.4
Hillsborough County	41.5	63.6	63.5	52.3	42.7	42.9	59.0	30.0
Los Angeles	73.6	77.5	85.6	68.7	54.0	62.0	67.0	37.8
Memphis	39.0	41.4	27.0	69.9	61.8	64.0	77.6	53.9
Miami	39.0	45.2	64.7	62.3	41.7	35.8	56.2	29.2
Orange County	35.7	62.6	71.8	54.6	37.7	60.5	55.5	25.8
Philadelphia	24.9	33.8	17.5	52.7	32.6	40.6	54.8	60.5
San Diego	30.0	60.5	48.4	87.4	73.1	78.0	62.9	30.2
San Francisco	67.6	64.7	76.5	60.6	60.6	44.1	60.6	29.4
Local Median	**41.1**	**60.1**	**49.5**	**65.0**	**53.0**	**61.0**	**61.8**	**32.4**
Local Range	**24.9 – 73.6**	**21.7 – 77.5**	**17.5 – 85.6**	**52.3 – 89.8**	**32.6 – 73.1**	**35.8 – 78.0**	**49.7 – 90.2**	**25.8 – 82.2**

* Survey did not include schools from the New York City Department of Education.

TABLE 22. Percentage of All Schools in Which the Lead Health Education Teacher Wanted to Receive Staff Development on Specific Topics, Selected U.S. Sites: School Health Profiles, Lead Health Education Teacher Surveys, 2006

Site	Teaching students with physical, medical, or cognitive disabilities	Teaching students of various cultural backgrounds	Teaching students with limited English proficiency	Using interactive teaching methods	Encouraging family or community involvement	Teaching skills for behavior change	Classroom management techniques	Assessing or evaluating students in health education
STATE SURVEYS								
Alabama	65.9	55.7	54.8	63.4	65.2	72.1	68.8	68.5
Alaska	60.2	54.7	49.9	58.2	62.5	71.3	65.9	62.5
Arizona	61.7	59.6	56.7	56.5	64.9	69.3	66.8	62.5
Arkansas	69.5	60.6	60.3	64.2	70.0	74.1	73.7	78.0
Connecticut	65.5	62.5	54.7	71.5	70.5	77.9	71.4	77.3
Delaware	72.9	64.1	64.8	67.1	67.0	80.3	68.3	81.8
Florida	64.6	60.3	55.2	64.1	66.5	77.1	68.9	68.0
Georgia	65.1	58.3	59.1	63.2	68.7	73.0	67.3	74.4
Hawaii	72.5	66.8	65.0	66.7	69.0	76.8	66.0	78.0
Idaho	67.2	58.5	55.5	57.8	61.0	72.4	70.5	70.2
Iowa	57.4	46.9	42.7	46.9	60.8	68.6	62.1	60.3
Kansas	56.3	42.3	38.7	55.1	63.9	72.8	64.5	68.6
Maine	55.5	36.5	35.0	54.9	55.9	70.8	64.8	58.6
Massachusetts	69.5	64.6	56.5	72.1	70.8	81.6	73.4	80.7
Michigan	62.1	59.7	46.3	60.7	63.0	72.8	63.2	64.9
Mississippi	63.9	63.8	60.6	63.5	67.1	73.6	70.5	72.6
Missouri	61.3	50.8	44.7	61.4	66.6	71.2	66.2	69.0
Montana	61.5	43.7	34.9	60.9	62.3	79.4	74.0	71.1
Nebraska	49.8	47.3	38.0	44.7	53.6	65.2	64.6	60.8
New Hampshire	64.9	53.4	47.4	67.1	68.2	79.6	70.7	77.1
New York*	68.7	58.0	53.5	69.9	69.9	85.7	73.7	83.2
North Carolina	69.6	63.0	63.3	59.9	63.6	72.7	67.3	68.3
North Dakota	56.0	41.4	30.7	46.3	56.9	73.3	58.9	60.9
Oregon	52.2	50.5	50.4	55.5	58.6	70.1	58.6	63.0
Pennsylvania	71.2	59.3	52.0	70.6	72.4	81.9	75.7	75.8
Rhode Island	68.7	52.8	49.4	66.6	61.6	81.3	68.8	82.4
South Carolina	64.0	59.4	60.4	59.1	64.1	71.8	63.3	72.5
South Dakota	50.1	41.8	31.1	51.8	57.0	68.5	65.2	60.8
Tennessee	72.3	62.3	60.4	62.1	65.9	77.4	73.1	70.2
Texas	61.8	58.4	56.9	63.3	63.2	69.3	63.8	62.2
Utah	63.6	59.9	57.6	66.7	60.4	79.1	69.2	68.4
Vermont	54.1	44.7	34.3	54.8	61.7	68.8	52.4	65.3
Virginia	62.3	53.8	54.1	52.3	53.8	69.3	62.3	66.4
West Virginia	59.9	45.3	42.2	61.1	64.6	72.5	66.8	68.9
State Median	**63.8**	**58.2**	**53.8**	**61.3**	**64.0**	**72.8**	**67.1**	**68.8**
State Range	**49.8 - 72.9**	**36.5 - 66.8**	**30.7 - 65.0**	**44.7 - 72.1**	**53.6 - 72.4**	**65.2 - 85.7**	**52.4 - 75.7**	**58.6 - 83.2**

TABLE 22. Percentage of All Schools in Which the Lead Health Education Teacher Wanted to Receive Staff Development on Specific Topics, Selected U.S. Sites: School Health Profiles, Lead Health Education Teacher Surveys, 2006 *(continued)*

Site	Teaching students with physical, medical, or cognitive disabilities	Teaching students of various cultural backgrounds	Teaching students with limited English proficiency	Using interactive teaching methods	Encouraging family or community involvement	Teaching skills for behavior change	Classroom management techniques	Assessing or evaluating students in health education
LOCAL SURVEYS								
Charlotte-Mecklenburg County	71.8	74.3	69.1	64.1	72.0	78.9	74.5	77.0
Chicago	74.3	66.6	60.2	70.1	76.1	78.7	81.3	71.9
Dallas	53.8	71.2	63.5	65.4	72.5	87.8	69.2	55.8
District of Columbia	77.3	77.3	65.7	73.2	76.8	80.7	80.0	74.1
Hillsborough County	45.2	43.6	43.4	46.5	53.0	63.2	58.0	48.9
Los Angeles	62.7	61.5	65.7	66.1	71.7	78.3	74.1	80.0
Memphis	90.2	82.0	81.4	81.9	87.7	90.7	86.5	91.8
Miami	72.9	67.1	54.4	71.3	72.9	77.9	76.7	67.1
Orange County	59.9	51.3	42.7	59.6	50.7	74.5	72.7	62.6
Philadelphia	81.6	78.0	75.5	78.2	75.9	91.0	82.5	73.5
San Diego	80.3	85.8	71.6	77.0	75.6	87.8	89.3	64.7
San Francisco	59.4	65.6	54.8	61.3	71.9	67.8	67.7	78.8
Local Median	**72.4**	**69.2**	**64.6**	**68.1**	**72.7**	**78.8**	**75.6**	**72.7**
Local Range	**45.2 - 90.2**	**43.6 - 85.8**	**42.7 - 81.4**	**46.5 - 81.9**	**50.7 - 87.7**	**63.2 - 91.0**	**58.0 - 89.3**	**48.9 - 91.8**

* Survey did not include schools from the New York City Department of Education.

TABLE 23. Percentage of All Schools That Required Physical Education in Any of Grades 6–12; the Percentage That Required Students to Take Only One Course or Two or More Courses; Among Schools That Required a Physical Education Course, the Percentage That Required Students Who Fail a Required Physical Education Course to Repeat It; and the Percentage of All Schools in Which a Newly Hired Physical Education Teacher is Required to be Certified* in Physical Education, Selected U.S. Sites: School Health Profiles, Principal Surveys, 2006

Site	Required physical education	Required only one physical education course	Required two or more physical education courses	Required students who fail a required physical education course to repeat it†	Newly hired physical education teacher required to be certified in physical education
STATE SURVEYS					
Alabama	98.0	36.6	60.1	62.1	99.2
Alaska	86.1	19.9	65.3	80.6	35.0
Arizona	73.1	31.8	39.1	39.6	67.9
Arkansas	99.2	36.8	62.0	73.1	97.7
Connecticut	100.0	16.7	82.4	48.7	97.9
Delaware	94.1	18.2	75.7	51.4	95.5
Florida	79.1	26.6	51.4	61.9	93.1
Georgia	85.5	41.9	42.9	56.6	98.3
Hawaii	93.1	35.3	57.6	66.5	85.3
Idaho	95.8	17.7	77.5	53.1	94.3
Illinois	100.0	11.7	88.0	40.8	98.2
Iowa	93.8	8.7	84.9	62.2	96.7
Kansas	98.8	37.6	60.6	58.5	98.8
Maine	98.8	23.0	75.0	46.2	95.9
Massachusetts	95.2	15.4	79.3	37.9	95.7
Michigan	90.0	35.2	54.1	55.3	97.3
Mississippi	36.8	19.0	14.4	64.6	97.8
Missouri	99.0	27.3	70.6	60.2	98.0
Montana	99.3	10.0	89.3	63.5	94.1
Nebraska	99.6	16.0	83.6	66.1	95.9
New Hampshire	97.7	18.0	78.4	43.4	99.5
New York‡	100.0	10.3	89.7	60.5	100.0
North Carolina	97.3	42.7	54.6	46.2	96.5
North Dakota	100.0	9.7	90.3	77.2	94.8
Oregon	97.3	18.7	78.1	51.2	85.4
Pennsylvania	98.4	11.5	86.9	56.2	97.7
Rhode Island	100.0	11.9	88.1	53.0	98.8
South Carolina	98.0	47.4	50.1	53.1	99.2
South Dakota	78.1	14.3	61.5	38.5	92.4
Tennessee	83.0	35.6	44.4	42.1	96.5
Texas	95.2	16.3	78.5	60.8	98.9
Utah	99.4	4.8	94.6	60.3	98.5
Vermont	97.1	10.5	85.9	49.6	98.6
Virginia	93.2	6.5	83.7	52.0	96.1
Washington	96.3	6.2	88.8	55.8	89.6
West Virginia	99.4	36.2	62.7	46.4	99.5
State Median	**97.3**	**18.1**	**76.6**	**55.6**	**97.0**
State Range	**36.8 - 100.0**	**4.8 - 47.4**	**14.4 - 94.6**	**37.9 - 80.6**	**35.0 - 100.0**

TABLE 23. Percentage of All Schools That Required Physical Education in Any of Grades 6–12; the Percentage That Required Students to Take Only One Course or Two or More Courses; Among Schools That Required a Physical Education Course, the Percentage That Required Students Who Fail a Required Physical Education Course to Repeat It; and the Percentage of All Schools in Which a Newly Hired Physical Education Teacher is Required to be Certified* in Physical Education, Selected U.S. Sites: School Health Profiles, Principal Surveys, 2006 *(continued)*

Site	Required physical education	Required only one physical education course	Required two or more physical education courses	Required students who fail a required physical education course to repeat it†	Newly hired physical education teacher required to be certified in physical education
LOCAL SURVEYS					
Charlotte-Mecklenburg County	100.0	34.0	66.0	43.8	97.7
Chicago	94.5	41.0	49.1	26.4	97.8
Dallas	98.0	16.1	81.9	59.1	100.0
District of Columbia	91.1	34.7	56.1	73.1	96.0
Hillsborough County	96.6	15.3	79.5	49.3	100.0
Los Angeles	98.7	4.7	93.9	45.3	98.7
Memphis	81.2	47.3	30.9	54.8	100.0
Miami	65.7	32.7	31.9	82.7	98.9
Orange County	44.0	12.4	31.6	78.8	96.9
Philadelphia	96.9	44.6	51.4	34.5	96.9
San Diego	96.6	8.9	87.7	57.3	100.0
San Francisco	93.7	22.3	68.2	37.9	90.6
Local Median	**95.6**	**27.5**	**61.1**	**52.1**	**98.3**
Local Range	**44.0 - 100.0**	**4.7 - 47.3**	**30.9 - 93.9**	**26.4 - 82.7**	**90.6 - 100.0**

* Certification, licensure, or endorsement by the state.
† Among schools that required physical education.
‡ Survey did not include schools from the New York City Department of Education.

TABLE 24. Percentage of Schools That Taught a Required Physical Education Course in Each Grade,* Selected U.S. Sites: School Health Profiles, Principal Surveys, 2006

Site	Grade 6	Grade 7	Grade 8	Grade 9	Grade 10	Grade 11	Grade 12
STATE SURVEYS							
Alabama	91.8	94.6	94.0	83.3	48.4	46.8	45.9
Alaska	60.3	64.1	63.4	71.3	65.0	47.5	40.8
Arizona	58.8	60.8	57.0	44.8	25.8	21.1	19.4
Arkansas	91.0	89.4	81.9	91.7	63.7	59.9	59.7
Connecticut	95.6	95.0	94.9	94.3	91.3	76.3	65.0
Delaware	80.0	81.5	82.9	76.3	58.7	21.2	18.7
Florida	60.0	59.4	58.8	59.5	47.0	36.1	34.1
Georgia	69.6	70.0	70.3	70.7	25.0	21.9	21.3
Hawaii	71.3	76.3	69.2	80.9	40.4	18.5	15.6
Idaho	83.2	88.0	82.8	54.9	58.9	39.2	36.2
Illinois	98.9	99.1	99.0	97.9	97.2	96.5	94.3
Iowa	87.1	90.0	89.9	87.8	88.0	87.5	87.5
Kansas	91.3	87.7	85.4	90.6	17.0	7.1	7.1
Maine	95.9	95.4	94.3	88.7	74.3	28.0	26.5
Massachusetts	89.7	91.0	91.2	85.0	77.6	57.3	52.4
Michigan	75.7	76.8	68.6	73.3	37.3	26.5	25.9
Mississippi	9.9	7.8	9.2	23.3	20.9	17.9	17.3
Missouri	92.6	95.3	95.3	90.4	46.9	27.9	29.1
Montana	94.8	95.1	96.8	98.8	94.5	12.8	11.5
Nebraska	93.8	96.1	96.1	87.7	46.7	18.6	16.0
New Hampshire	94.1	94.0	94.0	88.7	66.8	43.8	39.3
New York†	100.0	100.0	100.0	98.9	98.9	98.9	98.9
North Carolina	94.3	95.1	93.6	90.7	20.7	14.6	14.7
North Dakota	98.8	100.0	100.0	94.7	72.5	28.6	22.7
Oregon	92.5	91.5	91.6	87.3	66.2	35.8	31.1
Pennsylvania	95.4	97.0	97.0	92.8	92.3	88.7	82.4
Rhode Island	100.0	100.0	100.0	100.0	97.6	100.0	97.5
South Carolina	94.7	94.4	94.4	93.1	41.9	41.0	41.4
South Dakota	58.4	70.1	68.6	37.4	12.8	7.7	11.0
Tennessee	70.0	70.9	69.7	56.3	20.7	12.5	13.9
Texas	87.9	83.5	71.5	88.5	87.8	61.0	59.7
Utah	96.7	98.2	97.3	90.8	90.7	69.7	48.6
Vermont	92.2	94.8	94.8	88.6	80.3	53.8	50.1
Virginia	80.9	81.1	68.7	82.4	81.2	5.4	5.4
Washington	87.6	90.7	89.3	79.9	74.5	46.8	41.6
West Virginia	96.3	96.1	96.1	86.2	46.4	20.4	19.2
State Median	**91.6**	**91.3**	**91.4**	**87.8**	**64.4**	**36.0**	**32.6**
State Range	**9.9 - 100.0**	**7.8 - 100.0**	**9.2 - 100.0**	**23.3 - 100.0**	**12.8 - 98.9**	**5.4 - 100.0**	**5.4 - 98.9**

TABLE 24. Percentage of Schools That Taught a Required Physical Education Course in Each Grade,* Selected U.S. Sites: School Health Profiles, Principal Surveys, 2006 *(continued)*

Site	Grade 6	Grade 7	Grade 8	Grade 9	Grade 10	Grade 11	Grade 12
LOCAL SURVEYS							
Charlotte-Mecklenburg County	100.0	100.0	100.0	100.0	27.3	18.2	18.2
Chicago	87.1	88.0	87.9	64.2	63.2	19.3	16.0
Dallas	90.0	92.6	96.3	95.8	91.5	77.4	77.4
District of Columbia	64.7	56.8	54.4	87.4	82.1	19.6	19.6
Hillsborough County	83.4	87.1	87.1	72.3	72.3	47.8	47.8
Los Angeles	97.8	97.8	97.8	93.7	93.7	23.2	19.9
Memphis	53.9	60.3	63.4	67.1	21.2	19.3	19.3
Miami	30.9	26.0	21.7	50.2	42.8	17.3	17.6
Orange County	14.3	14.3	14.3	38.3	33.7	20.2	20.2
Philadelphia	91.0	90.1	90.1	63.9	83.1	68.2	60.2
San Diego	92.8	93.5	93.5	90.9	80.6	20.8	20.8
San Francisco	85.6	86.2	86.2	78.4	76.9	41.7	41.7
Local Median	**86.4**	**87.6**	**87.5**	**75.4**	**74.6**	**20.5**	**20.1**
Local Range	**14.3 - 100.0**	**14.3 - 100.0**	**14.3 - 100.0**	**38.3 - 100.0**	**21.2 - 93.7**	**17.3 - 77.4**	**16.0 - 77.4**

* Among schools with students in that grade.
† Survey did not include schools from the New York City Department of Education.

TABLE 25a. Among Schools That Required a Physical Education Course for Students in Any of Grades 6–12, the Percentage That Allowed Students to be Exempted from Taking a Required Physical Education Course for Specific Reasons, Selected U.S. Sites: School Health Profiles, Principal Surveys, 2006

Site	Religious reasons	Long-term physical or medical disability	Cognitive disability	Enrollment in other courses	Participation in school sports	Participation in other school activities*
STATE SURVEYS						
Alabama	23.0	63.1	18.1	7.6	17.5	38.2
Alaska	34.4	78.4	27.5	22.4	35.0	9.6
Arizona	52.8	86.1	34.8	18.8	13.6	25.8
Arkansas	32.8	75.3	28.6	16.5	44.4	15.7
Connecticut	33.0	87.2	12.9	5.5	2.9	0.4
Delaware	30.6	77.5	20.0	8.2	4.9	8.2
Florida	44.7	75.3	36.7	43.1	35.2	56.9
Georgia	38.0	77.1	31.2	30.7	3.8	36.0
Hawaii	40.0	85.0	36.5	18.4	1.9	10.4
Idaho	38.7	81.6	38.1	22.2	9.6	8.0
Illinois	47.1	85.7	25.8	24.1	32.1	22.4
Iowa	53.6	79.4	27.5	40.0	17.5	10.7
Kansas	47.7	79.8	34.6	9.9	5.8	3.9
Maine	34.0	83.3	21.8	15.7	3.9	2.6
Massachusetts	42.9	89.2	24.3	13.8	4.5	7.1
Michigan	42.8	87.9	35.0	15.1	15.2	28.0
Mississippi	64.5	79.7	59.8	48.7	57.4	51.6
Missouri	37.7	76.9	26.8	15.2	2.5	6.8
Montana	28.7	85.3	23.5	10.7	0.7	2.8
Nebraska	32.5	77.3	29.9	13.3	3.6	3.4
New Hampshire	33.2	81.1	18.0	16.0	12.0	7.3
New York†	16.6	65.5	11.5	1.4	10.9	0.3
North Carolina	34.1	68.4	18.7	11.2	1.4	9.6
North Dakota	20.4	64.9	21.1	10.6	0.6	1.2
Oregon	55.6	89.4	36.5	25.3	12.1	10.9
Pennsylvania	36.4	83.9	21.2	6.7	2.8	3.9
Rhode Island	29.7	88.1	15.6	0.0	2.5	0.0
South Carolina	47.9	82.2	31.4	21.4	3.1	52.5
South Dakota	22.4	69.9	30.4	11.2	5.0	2.4
Tennessee	45.2	79.7	37.9	12.7	4.6	36.7
Texas	35.7	79.2	37.1	16.9	75.4	56.8
Utah	44.7	92.7	51.6	17.3	29.3	10.4
Vermont	33.5	77.4	19.9	9.5	20.2	4.0
Virginia	40.9	79.5	28.7	11.4	0.5	6.8
Washington	61.5	89.7	36.8	34.3	35.6	20.8
West Virginia	16.3	70.2	15.0	8.0	0.5	4.5
State Median	**37.1**	**79.7**	**28.1**	**15.2**	**5.4**	**8.9**
State Range	**16.3 – 64.5**	**63.1 – 92.7**	**11.5 – 59.8**	**0.0 – 48.7**	**0.5 – 75.4**	**0.0 – 56.9**

TABLE 25a. Among Schools That Required a Physical Education Course for Students in Any of Grades 6–12, the Percentage That Allowed Students to be Exempted from Taking a Required Physical Education Course for Specific Reasons, Selected U.S. Sites: School Health Profiles, Principal Surveys, 2006 *(continued)*

Site	Religious reasons	Long-term physical or medical disability	Cognitive disability	Enrollment in other courses	Participation in school sports	Participation in other school activities*
LOCAL SURVEYS						
Charlotte-Mecklenburg County	37.3	69.2	12.7	15.0	5.0	19.5
Chicago	53.5	75.4	19.0	5.1	2.5	10.6
Dallas	33.3	79.3	47.2	12.8	53.9	64.3
District of Columbia	40.1	79.4	22.7	21.9	0.0	17.3
Hillsborough County	47.6	83.4	38.2	49.0	34.6	61.1
Los Angeles	27.5	73.8	16.3	5.8	42.8	33.4
Memphis	50.6	65.7	33.8	10.2	0.0	56.2
Miami	35.7	75.2	47.1	32.9	32.4	45.7
Orange County	55.0	47.9	42.3	31.0	73.2	64.8
Philadelphia	67.9	90.0	31.2	14.1	3.3	7.7
San Diego	32.2	92.6	40.1	16.8	49.3	50.2
San Francisco	48.3	87.3	26.3	7.0	13.9	20.9
Local Median	**43.9**	**77.4**	**32.5**	**14.6**	**23.2**	**39.6**
Local Range	**27.5 – 67.9**	**47.9 – 92.6**	**12.7 – 47.2**	**5.1 – 49.0**	**0.0 – 73.2**	**7.7 – 64.8**

* Such as ROTC, marching band, chorus, or cheerleading.
† Survey did not include schools from the New York City Department of Education.

TABLE 25b. Among Schools That Required a Physical Education Course for Students in Any of Grades 6–12, the Percentage That Allowed Students to be Exempted from Taking a Required Physical Education Course for Specific Reasons, Selected U.S. Sites: School Health Profiles, Principal Surveys, 2006

Site	Participation in community sports activities	High physical fitness competency test score	Participation in vocational training	Participation in community service activities	Could not be exempted from a required physical education course for certain reasons*
STATE SURVEYS					
Alabama	0.4	1.1	7.2	0.8	55.9
Alaska	13.4	7.1	6.2	4.5	49.5
Arizona	5.4	1.3	5.1	4.1	59.3
Arkansas	2.9	2.5	4.5	2.1	46.9
Connecticut	1.4	0.5	1.2	0.4	90.2
Delaware	1.7	0.0	1.6	1.6	79.7
Florida	3.6	12.4	11.3	5.0	21.1
Georgia	0.8	1.0	5.1	2.5	50.4
Hawaii	1.9	0.0	0.0	0.0	70.7
Idaho	4.5	1.0	3.7	1.5	64.8
Illinois	3.5	0.6	5.7	0.4	54.5
Iowa	1.3	0.8	8.3	1.7	50.5
Kansas	0.9	0.0	2.1	1.7	80.5
Maine	1.8	0.4	2.3	1.2	79.8
Massachusetts	2.7	0.2	2.5	1.2	77.0
Michigan	2.0	1.0	2.8	0.7	58.0
Mississippi	7.2	14.3	25.7	11.0	21.7
Missouri	0.3	0.0	1.7	0.3	80.5
Montana	1.1	0.7	1.1	1.1	88.5
Nebraska	0.0	0.0	1.0	0.9	81.1
New Hampshire	3.6	0.0	1.2	1.3	71.9
New York†	2.1	0.3	0.5	0.3	86.3
North Carolina	1.0	0.0	0.7	0.4	82.8
North Dakota	0.0	0.8	0.0	1.3	87.3
Oregon	11.6	3.2	5.1	3.9	63.1
Pennsylvania	2.3	2.1	6.3	1.0	82.7
Rhode Island	1.2	0.0	2.4	0.0	95.2
South Carolina	1.7	0.8	2.1	0.9	38.7
South Dakota	0.6	0.6	1.2	1.2	82.3
Tennessee	0.4	0.7	2.9	1.6	54.9
Texas	16.8	2.1	18.1	1.9	17.0
Utah	3.8	17.4	1.4	0.5	44.7
Vermont	7.5	0.0	3.2	3.1	72.1
Virginia	4.2	0.0	0.9	0.4	80.5
Washington	16.3	2.0	4.3	0.8	35.8
West Virginia	0.5	1.1	1.8	0.5	90.7
State Median	**2.0**	**0.8**	**2.5**	**1.2**	**71.3**
State Range	**0.0 – 16.8**	**0.0 – 17.4**	**0.0 – 25.7**	**0.0 – 11.0**	**17.0 – 95.2**

TABLE 25b. Among Schools That Required a Physical Education Course for Students in Any of Grades 6–12, the Percentage That Allowed Students to be Exempted from Taking a Required Physical Education Course for Specific Reasons, Selected U.S. Sites: School Health Profiles, Principal Surveys, 2006 *(continued)*

Site	Participation in community sports activities	High physical fitness competency test score	Participation in vocational training	Participation in community service activities	Could not be exempted from a required physical education course for certain reasons*
LOCAL SURVEYS					
Charlotte-Mecklenburg County	5.0	0.0	2.6	2.6	70.7
Chicago	3.1	0.5	1.0	2.0	83.6
Dallas	10.6	6.3	23.8	2.1	31.4
District of Columbia	0.0	0.0	0.0	3.8	68.0
Hillsborough County	2.1	14.7	2.5	0.0	16.8
Los Angeles	3.5	2.6	2.3	1.2	48.6
Memphis	0.0	2.7	2.4	0.0	34.3
Miami	2.0	13.4	7.4	1.8	29.4
Orange County	0.0	0.0	0.0	0.0	12.7
Philadelphia	3.6	3.5	1.2	2.1	76.2
San Diego	15.3	0.0	0.0	0.0	39.6
San Francisco	9.7	0.0	0.0	0.0	59.0
Local Median	**3.3**	**1.6**	**1.8**	**1.5**	**44.1**
Local Range	**0.0 - 15.3**	**0.0 - 14.7**	**0.0 - 23.8**	**0.0 - 3.8**	**12.7 - 83.6**

* These reasons included enrollment in other courses, participation in school sports, participation in other school activities, participation in community sports activities, high physical fitness competency test score, participation in vocational training, and participation in community service activities.

† Survey did not include schools from the New York City Department of Education.

TABLE 26. Percentage of All Schools That Supported or Promoted Walking or Biking to and from School, the Percentage of All Schools That Allowed Use of Their Physical Activity or Athletic Facilities* or Offered Opportunities for Students to Participate in Intramural Activities or Physical Activity Clubs, and Among Schools That Offered Opportunities for Students to Participate in Intramural Activities or Physical Activity Clubs, the Percentage That Provided Transportation Home,† Selected U.S. Sites: School Health Profiles, Principal Surveys, 2006

Site	Supported or promoted walking or biking to and from school	Allowed use of physical activity or athletic facilities	Offered intramural activities or physical activity clubs	Provided transportation home
STATE SURVEYS				
Alabama	24.8	75.5	44.6	10.3
Alaska	46.8	84.1	68.6	12.1
Arizona	62.9	64.0	71.3	51.7
Arkansas	37.7	82.7	38.1	12.1
Connecticut	31.1	89.7	80.9	52.2
Delaware	31.0	91.1	69.2	54.2
Florida	52.2	68.7	66.9	39.2
Georgia	28.1	82.6	60.7	23.9
Hawaii	42.9	73.4	90.1	14.1
Idaho	45.9	95.1	63.5	16.8
Illinois	55.3	89.1	58.3	35.8
Iowa	53.2	90.2	44.7	32.0
Kansas	48.2	93.2	35.4	31.8
Maine	48.6	94.6	82.1	46.9
Massachusetts	45.2	88.6	87.0	44.8
Michigan	46.3	86.4	72.7	13.6
Mississippi	10.3	66.8	43.3	18.7
Missouri	41.4	92.0	58.2	25.5
Montana	58.5	93.9	60.4	16.1
Nebraska	53.2	95.9	40.8	30.9
New Hampshire	53.0	94.4	84.7	39.3
New York‡	46.8	97.0	88.7	76.5
North Carolina	26.7	88.9	65.5	22.7
North Dakota	49.9	86.5	42.9	31.6
Oregon	59.9	91.0	60.7	27.1
Pennsylvania	36.2	84.9	82.9	38.4
Rhode Island	36.3	80.3	77.3	67.4
South Carolina	35.6	81.3	59.8	18.2
South Dakota	57.4	91.4	35.8	17.1
Tennessee	26.1	78.5	60.0	12.1
Texas	38.3	85.9	41.4	37.5
Utah	59.9	96.8	74.2	27.3
Vermont	58.5	97.6	83.3	30.6
Virginia	29.2	95.2	68.6	56.6
Washington	50.9	90.7	65.2	48.2
West Virginia	23.4	93.9	65.7	24.2
State Median	**46.1**	**89.4**	**65.4**	**30.8**
State Range	**10.3 - 62.9**	**64.0 - 97.6**	**35.4 - 90.1**	**10.3 - 76.5**

TABLE 26. Percentage of All Schools That Supported or Promoted Walking or Biking to and from School, the Percentage of All Schools That Allowed Use of Their Physical Activity or Athletic Facilities* or Offered Opportunities for Students to Participate in Intramural Activities or Physical Activity Clubs, and Among Schools That Offered Opportunities for Students to Participate in Intramural Activities or Physical Activity Clubs, the Percentage That Provided Transportation Home,† Selected U.S. Sites: School Health Profiles, Principal Surveys, 2006 *(continued)*

Site	Supported or promoted walking or biking to and from school	Allowed use of physical activity or athletic facilities	Offered intramural activities or physical activity clubs	Provided transportation home
LOCAL SURVEYS				
Charlotte-Mecklenburg County	30.8	97.7	61.9	23.4
Chicago	51.7	58.6	93.6	19.0
Dallas	18.1	58.0	67.0	51.2
District of Columbia	39.3	63.7	93.2	20.8
Hillsborough County	44.9	82.5	81.4	15.5
Los Angeles	70.6	98.9	75.5	32.4
Memphis	37.6	67.2	71.0	14.9
Miami	51.6	66.6	92.0	52.0
Orange County	80.8	90.7	95.0	18.3
Philadelphia	35.1	64.4	92.3	14.7
San Diego	70.1	77.0	71.9	68.0
San Francisco	38.1	60.7	87.7	6.8
Local Median	**42.1**	**66.9**	**84.6**	**19.9**
Local Range	**18.1 - 80.8**	**58.0 - 98.9**	**61.9 - 95.0**	**6.8 - 68.0**

* For community-sponsored sports teams, classes, or lessons outside of school hours or when school is not in session.
† For students who participate in after-school intramural activities or physical activity clubs.
‡ Survey did not include schools from the New York City Department of Education.

TABLE 27. Percentage of All Schools That Served Lunch to Students, and Among Those Schools, the Percentage in Which Students Usually Had 20 or More Minutes to Eat Lunch Once They Were Seated, Selected U.S. Sites: School Health Profiles, Principal Surveys, 2006

Site	Served lunch to students	≥20 minutes to eat lunch*
STATE SURVEYS		
Alabama	100.0	81.3
Alaska	91.1	90.4
Arizona	88.9	80.7
Arkansas	100.0	88.2
Connecticut	99.5	77.1
Delaware	100.0	82.2
Florida	98.9	85.5
Georgia	99.6	84.8
Hawaii	96.8	81.3
Idaho	100.0	84.5
Illinois	99.7	85.5
Iowa	97.7	66.8
Kansas	99.6	78.3
Maine	99.3	67.4
Massachusetts	99.8	76.7
Michigan	99.2	84.1
Mississippi	100.0	73.4
Missouri	100.0	64.7
Montana	99.2	85.2
Nebraska	99.2	83.6
New Hampshire	99.5	67.8
New York†	99.7	87.9
North Carolina	100.0	80.6
North Dakota	97.6	78.4
Oregon	99.6	83.3
Pennsylvania	98.4	89.5
Rhode Island	100.0	82.1
South Carolina	100.0	83.7
South Dakota	98.9	67.9
Tennessee	99.3	85.7
Texas	99.8	86.6
Utah	99.5	89.0
Vermont	100.0	68.2
Virginia	99.7	76.5
Washington	96.5	86.7
West Virginia	99.4	95.9
State Median	**99.6**	**82.8**
State Range	**88.9 - 100.0**	**64.7 - 95.9**

TABLE 27. Percentage of All Schools That Served Lunch to Students, and Among Those Schools, the Percentage in Which Students Usually Had 20 or More Minutes to Eat Lunch Once They Were Seated, Selected U.S. Sites: School Health Profiles, Principal Surveys, 2006 *(continued)*

Site	Served lunch to students	≥20 minutes to eat lunch*
LOCAL SURVEYS		
Charlotte-Mecklenburg County	100.0	64.2
Chicago	99.6	58.5
Dallas	98.0	67.4
District of Columbia	96.0	94.0
Hillsborough County	100.0	62.2
Los Angeles	100.0	81.8
Memphis	100.0	76.5
Miami	100.0	92.3
Orange County	100.0	74.5
Philadelphia	99.2	84.0
San Diego	100.0	80.5
San Francisco	100.0	94.4
Local Median	**100.0**	**78.5**
Local Range	**96.0 – 100.0**	**58.5 - 94.4**

* Among schools that served lunch to students.
† Survey did not include schools from the New York City Department of Education.

TABLE 28a. Percentage of All Schools That Allowed Students to Purchase Snack Foods or Beverages from One or More Vending Machines or at the School Store, Canteen, or Snack Bar, and That Allowed Students to Purchase Less Nutritious and More Nutritious Snack Foods and Beverages, Selected U.S. Sites: School Health Profiles, Principal Surveys, 2006

		Less Nutritious Foods and Beverages					
Site	Allowed students to purchase snack foods or beverages	2% or whole milk (plain or flavored)	Chocolate candy	Other kinds of candy	Salty snacks that are not low in fat*	Soda pop or fruit drinks that are not 100% juice	Sports drinks
STATE SURVEYS							
Alabama	86.7	32.3	32.3	37.4	45.4	69.7	81.9
Alaska	62.7	15.9	41.2	42.3	44.0	50.4	53.3
Arizona	68.6	27.1	32.8	36.2	40.0	43.1	58.8
Arkansas	70.7	33.5	23.5	26.3	26.2	64.2	58.5
Connecticut	71.8	49.5	21.2	25.8	41.2	39.5	57.3
Delaware	79.0	40.8	34.3	37.2	44.7	45.4	67.6
Florida	72.3	44.4	28.9	32.9	38.1	57.4	66.0
Georgia	87.1	40.3	53.9	56.9	59.4	73.3	82.6
Hawaii	61.9	17.3	12.6	14.2	11.0	39.5	30.5
Idaho	93.4	44.8	65.5	67.4	63.7	82.5	90.2
Illinois	77.2	50.2	43.2	46.5	52.2	63.7	67.5
Iowa	87.9	45.3	46.6	54.4	48.3	74.9	81.3
Kansas	85.7	32.5	62.2	63.0	60.4	79.1	78.9
Maine	77.6	42.4	8.4	11.2	23.0	25.3	59.5
Massachusetts	77.5	50.9	18.2	23.8	38.7	37.4	59.1
Michigan	87.6	55.2	58.6	64.2	68.2	67.7	78.9
Mississippi	87.9	34.0	71.0	72.0	75.0	78.2	78.5
Missouri	87.1	50.2	50.8	54.9	60.9	74.2	76.2
Montana	87.3	23.9	52.2	55.2	49.9	71.3	85.3
Nebraska	86.0	37.8	44.9	46.1	46.4	78.3	81.3
New Hampshire	90.5	60.2	22.2	24.5	44.6	43.4	73.1
New York†	93.3	60.9	34.5	44.8	61.7	62.5	81.5
North Carolina	84.3	40.1	35.0	40.3	50.0	56.0	72.2
North Dakota	78.4	23.3	45.7	44.1	38.2	69.1	73.4
Oregon	78.6	35.9	49.9	55.1	55.6	62.0	70.9
Pennsylvania	76.9	48.8	39.0	43.0	46.9	50.7	62.3
Rhode Island	89.5	67.9	26.4	28.8	49.8	44.0	71.0
South Carolina	94.0	49.2	56.4	66.0	69.9	76.0	86.6
South Dakota	80.5	35.4	28.3	29.7	27.5	66.6	77.1
Tennessee	88.0	45.6	58.4	61.9	62.5	73.3	81.9
Texas	81.0	49.6	46.9	39.9	47.9	56.3	70.9
Utah	93.0	58.6	82.9	82.6	75.9	86.0	87.9
Vermont	75.5	54.4	13.4	15.7	36.5	39.3	56.3
Virginia	80.2	47.2	47.2	51.5	60.0	62.4	67.0
Washington	88.2	41.1	39.4	46.5	39.6	57.8	75.1
West Virginia	82.3	32.9	10.1	18.2	28.3	37.3	48.6
State Median	**83.3**	**43.4**	**40.3**	**43.6**	**47.4**	**62.5**	**72.7**
State Range	**61.9 - 94.0**	**15.9 - 67.9**	**8.4 - 82.9**	**11.2 - 82.6**	**11.0 - 75.9**	**25.3 - 86.0**	**30.5 - 90.2**

TABLE 28a. Percentage of All Schools That Allowed Students to Purchase Snack Foods or Beverages from One or More Vending Machines or at the School Store, Canteen, or Snack Bar, and That Allowed Students to Purchase Less Nutritious and More Nutritious Snack Foods and Beverages, Selected U.S. Sites: School Health Profiles, Principal Surveys, 2006 *(continued)*

		Less Nutritious Foods and Beverages					
Site	Allowed students to purchase snack foods or beverages	2% or whole milk (plain or flavored)	Chocolate candy	Other kinds of candy	Salty snacks that are not low in fat*	Soda pop or fruit drinks that are not 100% juice	Sports drinks
LOCAL SURVEYS							
Charlotte-Mecklenburg County	85.7	48.0	47.6	57.3	81.0	66.1	73.3
Chicago	31.5	16.1	4.0	5.7	4.4	9.8	18.0
Dallas	76.9	35.0	59.1	56.9	65.6	71.4	69.8
District of Columbia	64.0	16.1	18.3	22.3	18.3	37.1	35.1
Hillsborough County	88.6	53.4	27.1	32.3	51.1	69.4	84.3
Los Angeles	88.0	55.3	8.2	16.0	15.5	9.6	76.5
Memphis	77.7	30.2	53.3	56.8	52.5	67.5	67.0
Miami	86.1	57.8	52.2	59.3	63.4	71.9	80.1
Orange County	80.7	49.9	21.1	24.3	33.3	47.4	74.3
Philadelphia	61.4	28.5	9.9	12.6	24.3	12.9	25.8
San Diego	84.5	64.6	43.8	43.8	67.0	57.3	78.6
San Francisco	62.3	30.2	5.9	12.3	6.5	15.1	28.1
Local Median	**79.2**	**41.5**	**24.1**	**28.3**	**42.2**	**52.4**	**71.6**
Local Range	**31.5 - 88.6**	**16.1 - 64.6**	**4.0 - 59.1**	**5.7 - 59.3**	**4.4 - 81.0**	**9.6 - 71.9**	**18.0 - 84.3**

* Such as regular potato chips.
† Survey did not include schools from the New York City Department of Education.

TABLE 28b. Percentage of All Schools That Allowed Students to Purchase Snack Foods or Beverages from One or More Vending Machines or at the School Store, Canteen, or Snack Bar, and That Allowed Students to Purchase Less Nutritious and More Nutritious Snack Foods and Beverages, Selected U.S. Sites: School Health Profiles, Principal Surveys, 2006

	More Nutritious Foods and Beverages					
Site	1% or skim milk	100% fruit juice or vegetable juice	Bottled water	Fruits or vegetables, not juice	Low-fat baked goods*	Salty snacks that are low in fat†
STATE SURVEYS						
Alabama	33.3	71.5	84.4	17.5	71.6	76.7
Alaska	10.7	50.6	55.6	14.7	36.2	42.7
Arizona	26.3	44.7	64.4	24.9	39.7	50.2
Arkansas	27.6	48.7	66.6	14.6	30.8	35.1
Connecticut	50.1	57.8	69.1	39.4	47.7	58.5
Delaware	40.2	62.1	74.5	23.9	47.6	56.6
Florida	43.7	55.4	70.2	29.6	42.5	49.5
Georgia	36.9	65.3	85.9	15.2	49.7	58.1
Hawaii	16.3	41.0	60.3	6.6	9.8	12.5
Idaho	36.0	77.0	90.8	28.6	57.6	71.2
Illinois	40.4	62.0	73.7	34.0	49.2	57.8
Iowa	44.1	72.5	85.9	28.2	49.3	57.6
Kansas	26.2	62.0	80.0	19.5	56.9	66.2
Maine	47.5	68.6	74.9	32.2	46.1	53.2
Massachusetts	52.1	64.7	75.2	34.9	53.9	62.4
Michigan	48.7	68.9	84.4	43.4	56.2	70.8
Mississippi	27.1	54.3	83.3	18.2	53.2	72.1
Missouri	45.6	65.5	81.9	23.6	52.4	62.4
Montana	22.0	69.6	83.1	25.1	41.9	52.1
Nebraska	35.6	62.6	78.8	17.1	45.4	52.2
New Hampshire	60.1	78.6	89.7	43.7	65.6	73.2
New York‡	59.8	77.0	89.6	46.8	65.2	79.2
North Carolina	41.2	63.8	79.9	30.6	55.7	62.0
North Dakota	21.7	64.0	75.9	14.5	33.7	43.2
Oregon	35.4	64.4	76.3	30.3	51.2	63.4
Pennsylvania	47.6	65.2	74.8	32.8	53.8	61.8
Rhode Island	66.2	77.7	84.6	46.8	55.8	68.7
South Carolina	42.7	66.9	90.2	25.9	66.7	75.9
South Dakota	33.2	66.1	79.7	19.0	36.7	39.9
Tennessee	35.7	63.1	85.1	22.0	57.1	67.4
Texas	44.9	67.2	77.6	41.2	59.6	68.5
Utah	45.8	74.4	89.7	36.8	73.4	82.9
Vermont	55.1	64.6	71.2	38.4	43.8	55.9
Virginia	40.6	62.9	77.6	25.2	58.1	69.1
Washington	36.0	73.7	85.1	33.9	57.9	62.9
West Virginia	33.1	67.0	79.3	7.6	62.3	67.8
State Median	**40.3**	**65.0**	**79.5**	**27.1**	**52.8**	**62.2**
State Range	**10.7 - 66.2**	**41.0 - 78.6**	**55.6 - 90.8**	**6.6 - 46.8**	**9.8 - 73.4**	**12.5 - 82.9**

TABLE 28b. Percentage of All Schools That Allowed Students to Purchase Snack Foods or Beverages from One or More Vending Machines or at the School Store, Canteen, or Snack Bar, and That Allowed Students to Purchase Less Nutritious and More Nutritious Snack Foods and Beverages, Selected U.S. Sites: School Health Profiles, Principal Surveys, 2006 *(continued)*

	More Nutritious Foods and Beverages					
Site	1% or skim milk	100% fruit juice or vegetable juice	Bottled water	Fruits or vegetables, not juice	Low-fat baked goods*	Salty snacks that are low in fat†
LOCAL SURVEYS						
Charlotte-Mecklenburg County	50.4	71.7	81.0	41.0	69.2	81.0
Chicago	14.7	25.0	29.0	10.3	13.4	14.2
Dallas	21.8	43.9	72.1	19.7	45.8	56.7
District of Columbia	24.3	42.7	55.8	14.2	22.3	25.5
Hillsborough County	53.6	66.9	86.5	38.7	46.6	65.1
Los Angeles	56.7	75.9	86.6	43.6	66.5	67.8
Memphis	25.1	61.6	56.6	17.9	32.0	42.7
Miami	60.1	62.7	80.3	39.3	62.5	72.0
Orange County	44.2	53.2	78.2	32.6	51.9	55.7
Philadelphia	29.2	53.5	54.7	23.1	40.4	42.7
San Diego	46.1	67.1	78.6	58.8	56.6	72.4
San Francisco	36.7	52.2	61.2	39.6	45.7	46.1
Local Median	**40.5**	**57.6**	**75.2**	**35.7**	**46.2**	**56.2**
Local Range	**14.7 - 60.1**	**25.0 - 75.9**	**29.0 - 86.6**	**10.3 - 58.8**	**13.4 - 69.2**	**14.2 - 81.0**

* Such as cookies, crackers, cakes, pastries, or other low-fat baked goods.
† Such as pretzels, baked chips, or other low-fat chips.
‡ Survey did not include schools from the New York City Department of Education.

TABLE 29. Percentage of All Schools That Allowed Students to Purchase Candy; Snacks That are Not Low in Fat; Soda Pop, Sports Drinks, or Fruit Drinks That Are Not 100% Juice; or 2% or Whole Milk During Specific Times and the Percentage of Schools That Had a Policy Stating That Fruits and Vegetables Will Be Among the Foods Offered at School Settings,* Selected U.S. Sites: School Health Profiles, Principal Surveys, 2006

Site	Before classes begin in the morning	During any school hours when meals are not being served	During school lunch periods	Offered fruits or vegetables
STATE SURVEYS				
Alabama	28.9	45.3	13.9	38.0
Alaska	29.2	25.3	29.8	22.2
Arizona	38.8	28.2	34.9	24.6
Arkansas	30.8	25.5	34.6	35.5
Connecticut	21.6	20.3	32.6	27.0
Delaware	23.9	11.9	26.9	15.6
Florida	34.2	33.7	33.8	19.5
Georgia	41.0	36.6	44.4	11.1
Hawaii	20.2	16.7	3.9	21.0
Idaho	67.5	52.5	69.1	16.5
Illinois	42.3	23.0	45.6	9.9
Iowa	59.4	44.3	35.5	11.9
Kansas	60.9	39.5	39.9	11.2
Maine	21.3	13.0	18.5	35.5
Massachusetts	24.1	13.7	44.0	18.1
Michigan	52.3	28.9	64.3	11.9
Mississippi	28.9	50.0	11.9	17.6
Missouri	56.1	25.7	57.5	13.8
Montana	57.3	41.6	58.4	18.1
Nebraska	55.6	40.9	14.4	10.8
New Hampshire	38.6	29.2	37.6	19.9
New York†	35.3	30.1	45.7	14.4
North Carolina	27.2	22.8	22.4	17.2
North Dakota	52.7	32.9	28.8	21.6
Oregon	41.8	33.4	46.2	17.5
Pennsylvania	31.3	15.3	40.1	29.3
Rhode Island	34.7	16.9	58.4	24.4
South Carolina	38.6	30.3	63.2	14.9
South Dakota	54.3	46.8	22.7	16.8
Tennessee	32.3	46.2	22.2	14.6
Texas	31.3	29.1	34.8	29.6
Utah	72.5	56.6	81.3	20.2
Vermont	32.2	29.4	32.1	15.2
Virginia	33.9	23.4	31.3	11.1
Washington	43.4	33.1	43.8	27.6
West Virginia	25.4	26.2	11.6	29.8
State Median	**35.0**	**29.3**	**34.9**	**17.9**
State Range	**20.2 - 72.5**	**11.9 - 56.6**	**3.9 - 81.3**	**9.9 - 38.0**

TABLE 29. Percentage of All Schools That Allowed Students to Purchase Candy; Snacks That are Not Low in Fat; Soda Pop, Sports Drinks, or Fruit Drinks That Are Not 100% Juice; or 2% or Whole Milk During Specific Times and the Percentage of Schools That Had a Policy Stating That Fruits and Vegetables Will Be Among the Foods Offered at School Settings,* Selected U.S. Sites: School Health Profiles, Principal Surveys, 2006 *(continued)*

Site	Before classes begin in the morning	During any school hours when meals are not being served	During school lunch periods	Offered fruits or vegetables
LOCAL SURVEYS				
Charlotte-Mecklenburg County	31.8	16.9	48.6	21.4
Chicago	7.2	3.1	15.7	31.9
Dallas	38.8	28.1	47.4	19.9
District of Columbia	24.7	3.1	45.7	30.9
Hillsborough County	30.5	37.1	29.2	11.7
Los Angeles	18.0	5.7	19.4	28.2
Memphis	14.1	5.5	35.9	15.7
Miami	58.0	33.7	52.6	24.6
Orange County	39.1	39.1	37.8	8.7
Philadelphia	10.5	7.1	30.8	41.5
San Diego	34.3	19.3	72.3	21.6
San Francisco	11.9	2.9	18.4	62.3
Local Median	**27.6**	**12.0**	**36.9**	**23.1**
Local Range	**7.2 - 58.0**	**2.9 - 39.1**	**15.7 - 72.3**	**8.7 - 62.3**

* Such as student parties, after-school or extended day programs, or concession stands.
† Survey did not include schools from the New York City Department of Education.

TABLE 30. Percentage of All Schools That Had a Policy Prohibiting Tobacco Use and the Percentage That Prohibited All Tobacco Use in All Locations,* Selected U.S. Sites: School Health Profiles, Principal Surveys, 2006

Site	Had a policy prohibiting tobacco use	Prohibited all tobacco use in all locations
STATE SURVEYS		
Alabama	97.9	57.3
Alaska	94.3	26.8
Arizona	97.4	56.2
Arkansas	99.6	57.4
Connecticut	97.9	52.1
Delaware	100.0	56.4
Florida	95.4	40.4
Georgia	99.6	56.7
Hawaii	98.4	62.2
Idaho	99.1	44.2
Illinois	99.0	44.9
Iowa	98.0	25.3
Kansas	98.4	26.2
Maine	99.3	58.0
Massachusetts	98.4	59.2
Michigan	95.9	39.2
Mississippi	99.4	62.2
Missouri	98.3	24.0
Montana	100.0	53.8
Nebraska	99.6	31.6
New Hampshire	99.5	49.6
New York†	98.0	64.4
North Carolina	97.2	45.3
North Dakota	100.0	39.7
Oregon	98.9	58.4
Pennsylvania	98.8	53.9
Rhode Island	97.7	61.7
South Carolina	99.3	47.0
South Dakota	96.0	22.8
Tennessee	99.0	30.3
Texas	98.5	62.2
Utah	99.5	53.8
Vermont	100.0	63.1
Virginia	98.9	43.7
Washington	99.0	64.9
West Virginia	98.9	76.3
State Median	**98.9**	**53.8**
State Range	**94.3 - 100.0**	**22.8 - 76.3**

TABLE 30. Percentage of All Schools That Had a Policy Prohibiting Tobacco Use and the Percentage That Prohibited All Tobacco Use in All Locations,* Selected U.S. Sites: School Health Profiles, Principal Surveys, 2006 *(continued)*

Site	Had a policy prohibiting tobacco use	Prohibited all tobacco use in all locations
LOCAL SURVEYS		
Charlotte-Mecklenburg County	100.0	74.8
Chicago	84.0	36.4
Dallas	98.0	62.6
District of Columbia	94.2	41.0
Hillsborough County	92.6	15.5
Los Angeles	100.0	67.9
Memphis	98.3	50.3
Miami	96.6	53.3
Orange County	100.0	79.5
Philadelphia	95.5	34.1
San Diego	100.0	74.0
San Francisco	100.0	58.7
Local Median	**98.2**	**56.0**
Local Range	**84.0 - 100.0**	**15.5 - 79.5**

* Prohibited the use of all tobacco, including cigarettes, smokeless tobacco (i.e., chewing tobacco, snuff, or dip), cigars, and pipes; by students, faculty and school staff, and visitors; in school buildings, outside on school grounds (including parking lots and playing fields), on school buses or other vehicles used to transport students, and at off-campus, school-sponsored events.

† Survey did not include schools from the New York City Department of Education.

TABLE 31a. Among Schools with a Policy Prohibiting Tobacco Use, the Percentage of Schools That Sometimes, Almost Always, or Always Took Specific Actions When Students Were Caught Smoking Cigarettes, Selected U.S. Sites: School Health Profiles, Principal Surveys, 2006

Site	Informed parents or guardians	Referred to a school counselor	Referred to a school administrator	Encouraged to participate in an assistance, education, or cessation program	Required to participate in an assistance, education, or cessation program
STATE SURVEYS					
Alabama	96.8	69.0	97.5	39.3	14.8
Alaska	93.2	61.1	92.6	51.1	26.8
Arizona	96.8	68.8	95.9	58.2	29.6
Arkansas	99.2	67.8	98.8	44.0	23.5
Connecticut	97.3	83.2	96.5	64.6	29.2
Delaware	100.0	77.4	98.4	68.7	32.7
Florida	95.3	73.1	93.6	58.0	43.1
Georgia	99.2	69.6	98.9	41.7	19.9
Hawaii	98.3	88.6	96.6	75.1	40.0
Idaho	99.1	87.4	98.1	69.5	58.9
Illinois	98.4	71.5	97.1	49.2	23.6
Iowa	97.9	76.6	97.9	61.9	37.7
Kansas	98.4	76.4	97.0	48.5	25.0
Maine	98.8	86.1	98.4	76.0	46.4
Massachusetts	97.4	78.6	97.5	68.0	31.2
Michigan	95.0	72.1	95.5	59.9	30.6
Mississippi	98.9	57.1	98.9	30.4	10.3
Missouri	97.7	63.9	97.9	32.5	15.3
Montana	100.0	83.0	100.0	68.4	48.4
Nebraska	99.2	76.9	99.2	56.6	26.8
New Hampshire	99.4	85.0	98.9	73.2	39.9
New York*	97.7	85.8	97.7	71.1	32.6
North Carolina	96.7	73.4	96.7	55.9	42.6
North Dakota	99.2	77.5	98.3	60.4	28.2
Oregon	98.1	77.1	96.8	74.7	50.2
Pennsylvania	98.1	78.6	97.4	71.6	41.0
Rhode Island	96.5	90.5	97.6	73.6	47.1
South Carolina	98.8	71.8	99.3	49.0	26.6
South Dakota	94.8	74.0	95.3	46.7	28.3
Tennessee	98.0	68.9	98.7	50.2	34.4
Texas	98.2	70.1	97.9	45.5	22.9
Utah	99.5	78.7	99.5	81.2	70.4
Vermont	98.6	92.1	98.6	76.5	56.9
Virginia	98.9	76.8	98.9	57.4	39.5
Washington	97.9	85.5	98.7	76.3	58.1
West Virginia	98.8	81.3	98.8	69.8	64.0
State Median	**98.3**	**76.9**	**97.9**	**60.2**	**32.7**
State Range	**93.2 - 100.0**	**57.1 - 92.1**	**92.6 - 100.0**	**30.3 - 81.2**	**10.3 - 70.4**

TABLE 31a. Among Schools with a Policy Prohibiting Tobacco Use, the Percentage of Schools That Sometimes, Almost Always, or Always Took Specific Actions When Students Were Caught Smoking Cigarettes, Selected U.S. Sites: School Health Profiles, Principal Surveys, 2006 *(continued)*

Site	Informed parents or guardians	Referred to a school counselor	Referred to a school administrator	Encouraged to participate in an assistance, education, or cessation program	Required to participate in an assistance, education, or cessation program
LOCAL SURVEYS					
Charlotte-Mecklenburg County	97.4	90.1	97.5	79.6	84.7
Chicago	82.5	66.2	81.1	38.7	18.2
Dallas	97.9	66.4	97.8	44.5	24.4
District of Columbia	93.7	74.7	93.7	51.4	46.1
Hillsborough County	92.3	65.6	92.2	48.9	31.0
Los Angeles	98.9	92.1	87.6	74.2	72.2
Memphis	98.3	84.4	98.3	65.1	54.6
Miami	96.5	93.0	95.4	72.3	38.2
Orange County	100.0	85.4	100.0	66.2	51.0
Philadelphia	94.1	78.0	88.4	50.7	23.2
San Diego	100.0	98.2	100.0	90.7	72.8
San Francisco	90.3	96.8	93.7	80.5	78.9
Local Median	**97.0**	**84.9**	**94.6**	**65.7**	**48.6**
Local Range	**82.5 - 100.0**	**65.6 - 98.2**	**81.1 - 100.0**	**38.7 - 90.7**	**18.2 - 84.7**

* Survey did not include schools from the New York City Department of Education.

TABLE 31b. Among Schools with a Policy Prohibiting Tobacco Use, the Percentage of Schools That Sometimes, Almost Always, or Always Took Specific Actions When Students Were Caught Smoking Cigarettes, Selected U.S. Sites: School Health Profiles, Principal Surveys, 2006

Site	Referred to legal authorities	Placed in detention	Given in-school suspension	Not allowed to participate in extracurricular activities or interscholastic sports	Suspended from school	Expelled from school	Reassigned to an alternative school
STATE SURVEYS							
Alabama	19.0	61.5	67.7	58.5	83.5	7.0	37.7
Alaska	51.8	55.8	54.7	76.8	72.2	6.5	1.6
Arizona	51.2	66.4	69.2	64.2	80.0	12.2	13.7
Arkansas	31.2	62.4	79.1	64.2	75.6	11.3	20.0
Connecticut	28.4	67.0	70.1	63.4	78.3	7.5	3.6
Delaware	18.9	62.5	75.8	54.2	82.9	9.4	10.8
Florida	59.8	59.2	66.8	49.9	72.2	5.3	13.7
Georgia	19.9	58.4	83.5	56.9	72.9	9.4	18.0
Hawaii	17.3	77.8	62.2	53.3	78.8	0.0	2.2
Idaho	95.5	67.8	71.9	92.4	82.2	15.5	11.2
Illinois	40.2	73.3	73.8	87.8	80.5	8.3	8.2
Iowa	78.8	59.9	74.8	94.2	66.4	4.8	2.9
Kansas	69.1	64.5	67.1	86.1	71.5	13.4	3.8
Maine	73.9	56.3	59.2	89.5	85.8	8.2	2.6
Massachusetts	22.2	70.4	60.9	65.3	75.1	1.6	1.6
Michigan	63.2	51.5	54.7	79.2	88.5	8.9	5.5
Mississippi	25.0	57.7	74.3	62.6	79.4	4.5	20.6
Missouri	41.7	70.1	80.6	74.8	72.6	7.9	9.0
Montana	83.9	70.8	71.7	92.3	78.1	9.2	2.7
Nebraska	56.1	75.6	81.1	93.4	73.9	11.4	5.0
New Hampshire	83.7	57.9	61.5	77.6	80.6	3.7	0.6
New York*	19.5	74.1	83.4	82.8	71.6	5.2	4.9
North Carolina	16.6	65.6	75.3	54.5	74.9	7.2	10.3
North Dakota	68.7	67.4	67.4	97.7	60.8	3.7	1.4
Oregon	66.7	62.8	68.8	76.3	79.8	17.1	14.8
Pennsylvania	74.2	53.1	67.3	69.5	67.6	5.9	6.3
Rhode Island	32.7	84.4	55.6	59.8	67.1	2.3	3.5
South Carolina	15.4	62.1	70.1	58.7	89.0	18.9	26.6
South Dakota	63.8	72.8	71.3	93.7	61.8	8.5	2.7
Tennessee	77.2	55.3	66.7	57.6	70.8	14.9	32.1
Texas	65.6	78.3	89.7	74.0	53.2	10.9	29.4
Utah	97.2	59.4	62.7	74.7	86.5	15.2	14.2
Vermont	65.7	54.7	74.8	80.1	73.6	5.0	4.4
Virginia	68.9	50.9	62.5	71.4	88.1	5.6	11.5
Washington	48.6	59.1	60.9	85.0	85.9	11.2	6.4
West Virginia	69.3	63.6	57.3	61.6	73.3	9.0	16.4
State Median	**58.0**	**62.7**	**69.0**	**74.4**	**75.4**	**8.3**	**7.3**
State Range	**15.4 - 97.2**	**50.9 - 84.4**	**54.7 - 89.7**	**49.9 - 97.7**	**53.2 - 89.0**	**0.6 - 18.9**	**0.6 - 37.7**

TABLE 31b. Among Schools with a Policy Prohibiting Tobacco Use, the Percentage of Schools That Sometimes, Almost Always, or Always Took Specific Actions When Students Were Caught Smoking Cigarettes, Selected U.S. Sites: School Health Profiles, Principal Surveys, 2006 *(continued)*

Site	Referred to legal authorities	Placed in detention	Given in-school suspension	Not allowed to participate in extracurricular activities or interscholastic sports	Suspended from school	Expelled from school	Reassigned to an alternative school
LOCAL SURVEYS							
Charlotte-Mecklenburg County	45.0	87.0	67.3	56.1	67.3	9.8	17.8
Chicago	25.3	65.4	64.9	51.5	70.0	7.0	4.7
Dallas	55.1	77.3	93.3	54.5	84.1	17.7	26.5
District of Columbia	35.1	68.2	61.6	57.1	76.9	17.6	31.6
Hillsborough County	75.4	57.4	72.1	36.9	75.2	1.9	3.4
Los Angeles	52.3	65.5	56.5	45.0	74.6	3.9	5.3
Memphis	53.3	64.3	75.9	60.0	92.8	22.3	22.7
Miami	37.3	67.8	85.8	51.7	70.2	10.5	17.4
Orange County	51.9	63.1	88.5	57.1	84.8	9.6	9.6
Philadelphia	19.3	79.5	73.2	64.0	74.9	5.6	10.9
San Diego	66.4	71.8	54.7	61.4	90.9	24.2	24.1
San Francisco	30.7	52.2	61.4	51.3	56.4	0.0	0.0
Local Median	**48.5**	**66.7**	**69.7**	**55.3**	**75.1**	**9.7**	**14.2**
Local Range	**19.3 - 75.4**	**52.2 - 87.0**	**54.7 - 93.3**	**36.9 - 64.0**	**56.4 - 92.8**	**0.0 - 24.2**	**0.0 - 31.6**

* Survey did not include schools from the New York City Department of Education.

TABLE 32. Among Schools with a Policy Prohibiting Tobacco Use, the Percentage of Schools That Had Procedures to Inform Specific Groups About the Tobacco Prevention Policy That Prohibits Their Use of Tobacco and a Policy to Inform Students' Families About the Rules Related to Tobacco Use by Students, Selected U.S. Sites: School Health Profiles, Principal Surveys, 2006

	Groups informed about policy prohibiting their use of tobacco			
Site	Students	Faculty and staff	Visitors	Informed students' families of rules related to tobacco use
STATE SURVEYS				
Alabama	99.6	98.8	92.2	98.9
Alaska	99.0	94.2	83.8	97.9
Arizona	98.4	95.4	87.3	97.2
Arkansas	99.7	99.3	96.2	100.0
Connecticut	98.8	93.4	76.4	98.8
Delaware	98.4	93.7	87.1	100.0
Florida	99.7	95.6	89.2	96.9
Georgia	99.7	97.6	83.8	97.8
Hawaii	100.0	97.6	89.8	98.7
Idaho	100.0	94.5	76.9	95.4
Illinois	98.1	94.3	82.5	96.9
Iowa	100.0	94.7	78.1	97.7
Kansas	98.4	93.5	77.1	97.9
Maine	99.3	98.2	87.3	98.5
Massachusetts	99.5	98.3	85.0	99.1
Michigan	99.0	95.4	81.0	97.6
Mississippi	100.0	97.6	92.5	98.3
Missouri	99.4	95.5	78.8	98.6
Montana	99.1	98.3	96.1	99.6
Nebraska	99.5	94.4	74.0	99.0
New Hampshire	98.9	95.9	85.6	98.2
New York*	99.7	98.6	93.3	99.4
North Carolina	99.7	98.6	89.1	99.0
North Dakota	100.0	95.9	87.9	98.7
Oregon	100.0	98.6	90.2	100.0
Pennsylvania	99.7	97.4	88.7	98.2
Rhode Island	97.6	96.5	83.9	95.2
South Carolina	99.1	97.5	87.2	98.7
South Dakota	98.9	90.6	77.8	96.7
Tennessee	99.7	97.5	91.0	99.3
Texas	99.5	97.6	89.6	96.8
Utah	100.0	96.0	74.7	98.6
Vermont	99.3	96.3	90.3	100.0
Virginia	100.0	98.9	92.7	99.6
Washington	99.3	95.6	90.0	98.9
West Virginia	100.0	99.4	96.6	100.0
State Median	**99.5**	**96.4**	**87.3**	**98.7**
State Range	**97.6 - 100.0**	**90.6 - 99.4**	**74.0 - 96.6**	**95.2 - 100.0**

TABLE 32. Among Schools with a Policy Prohibiting Tobacco Use, the Percentage of Schools That Had Procedures to Inform Specific Groups About the Tobacco Prevention Policy That Prohibits Their Use of Tobacco and a Policy to Inform Students' Families About the Rules Related to Tobacco Use by Students, Selected U.S. Sites: School Health Profiles, Principal Surveys, 2006 *(continued)*

	Groups informed about policy prohibiting their use of tobacco			
Site	Students	Faculty and staff	Visitors	Informed students' families of rules related to tobacco use
LOCAL SURVEYS				
Charlotte-Mecklenburg County	100.0	100.0	94.8	100.0
Chicago	96.9	96.4	85.2	92.8
Dallas	97.9	100.0	90.8	91.5
District of Columbia	95.8	81.3	75.9	92.5
Hillsborough County	97.8	81.6	69.5	100.0
Los Angeles	100.0	100.0	96.0	100.0
Memphis	98.0	98.0	89.4	94.6
Miami	98.8	96.4	86.7	93.0
Orange County	100.0	100.0	93.8	100.0
Philadelphia	98.0	93.8	86.6	96.0
San Diego	100.0	85.9	85.9	96.1
San Francisco	97.2	91.4	78.8	90.9
Local Median	**98.0**	**96.4**	**86.7**	**95.3**
Local Range	**95.8 - 100.0**	**81.3 - 100.0**	**69.5 - 96.0**	**90.9 - 100.0**

* Survey did not include schools from the New York City Department of Education.

TABLE 33. Percentage of All Schools That Prohibited Tobacco Advertising in Specific Locations, Through Sponsorship of School Events, or on Student Apparel or Merchandise, or Prohibited All Tobacco Advertising, Selected U.S. Sites: School Health Profiles, Principal Surveys, 2006

Site	In school building	On school grounds*	On school buses or other vehicles†	In school publications	Through sponsorship of school events	On tobacco brand-name apparel or merchandise‡	All tobacco advertising§
STATE SURVEYS							
Alabama	96.6	95.8	95.7	96.3	94.9	98.3	89.8
Alaska	96.4	94.8	95.4	94.1	90.4	84.7	75.8
Arizona	96.4	96.4	96.1	93.7	93.3	98.8	88.7
Arkansas	95.4	94.6	95.4	93.2	91.2	95.8	81.8
Connecticut	95.7	95.7	95.3	95.3	92.9	87.5	77.9
Delaware	100.0	100.0	98.5	98.5	92.7	85.3	78.0
Florida	96.7	95.4	95.0	96.0	95.2	97.0	87.7
Georgia	94.2	94.2	92.8	93.0	89.3	97.2	84.0
Hawaii	94.5	95.1	92.1	93.4	94.1	96.3	82.5
Idaho	96.6	95.1	96.1	94.1	95.5	98.6	89.4
Illinois	95.6	95.2	95.6	94.9	95.5	95.7	86.8
Iowa	95.3	94.0	93.6	93.7	92.2	96.5	86.5
Kansas	93.6	93.5	93.2	93.1	92.2	95.1	84.2
Maine	95.3	95.6	94.6	95.0	93.8	94.8	84.4
Massachusetts	94.2	93.6	93.3	93.1	91.5	79.1	69.5
Michigan	94.7	93.2	92.9	92.6	92.6	94.8	84.2
Mississippi	95.5	95.5	95.5	93.2	90.3	96.7	84.3
Missouri	92.1	91.4	91.3	91.5	91.5	95.3	80.5
Montana	98.4	98.1	98.0	98.0	95.9	96.5	91.6
Nebraska	93.6	92.3	91.8	93.2	92.5	98.4	84.6
New Hampshire	93.9	93.9	93.3	93.3	94.5	95.7	85.7
New York‖	93.3	92.4	92.7	93.0	95.0	82.6	71.8
North Carolina	93.2	92.2	92.2	92.2	89.8	84.7	71.5
North Dakota	93.7	93.2	92.3	93.7	94.6	96.7	87.3
Oregon	92.6	92.7	93.1	92.6	92.3	98.3	85.4
Pennsylvania	93.0	91.8	92.4	92.4	91.7	93.6	80.2
Rhode Island	95.4	96.5	95.3	94.1	89.5	78.2	68.8
South Carolina	97.2	97.2	96.4	95.4	93.9	90.7	82.1
South Dakota	92.2	90.8	92.2	90.6	91.5	98.5	85.5
Tennessee	95.6	93.9	94.6	93.1	92.0	95.4	83.0
Texas	95.4	94.9	94.8	93.8	92.1	98.4	86.6
Utah	95.9	94.0	95.0	93.9	93.7	98.9	87.0
Vermont	98.6	98.6	96.5	98.6	95.5	96.9	88.9
Virginia	95.4	94.3	94.6	94.9	93.1	91.2	81.3
Washington	98.4	97.8	96.3	95.4	94.0	94.1	84.8
West Virginia	95.8	95.3	95.4	93.8	91.5	95.5	84.9
State Median	**95.4**	**94.7**	**94.7**	**93.7**	**92.7**	**95.7**	**84.4**
State Range	**92.1 - 100.0**	**90.8 - 100.0**	**91.3 - 98.5**	**90.6 - 98.6**	**89.3 - 95.9**	**78.2 - 98.9**	**68.8 - 91.6**

TABLE 33. Percentage of All Schools That Prohibited Tobacco Advertising in Specific Locations, Through Sponsorship of School Events, or on Student Apparel or Merchandise, or Prohibited All Tobacco Advertising, Selected U.S. Sites: School Health Profiles, Principal Surveys, 2006 *(continued)*

Site	In school building	On school grounds*	On school buses or other vehicles†	In school publications	Through sponsorship of school events	On tobacco brand-name apparel or merchandise‡	All tobacco advertising§
LOCAL SURVEYS							
Charlotte-Mecklenburg County	95.2	95.2	95.2	95.2	80.8	80.9	68.9
Chicago	92.6	89.5	89.0	90.4	88.4	90.0	73.2
Dallas	91.7	91.7	89.7	89.5	87.9	97.9	79.2
District of Columbia	90.3	90.3	90.3	87.4	84.1	71.6	52.2
Hillsborough County	90.9	87.2	85.5	87.5	90.8	90.8	74.1
Los Angeles	97.8	97.8	97.8	95.7	94.3	94.5	85.3
Memphis	93.0	93.0	93.0	91.5	87.7	98.3	82.5
Miami	95.7	94.6	93.5	95.5	94.3	92.2	79.8
Orange County	91.3	88.2	84.7	88.8	97.5	97.5	80.1
Philadelphia	98.0	93.3	98.0	94.2	90.4	88.7	72.6
San Diego	100.0	100.0	98.2	98.2	92.8	100.0	91.0
San Francisco	94.4	91.6	91.6	91.6	97.1	85.3	79.2
Local Median	**93.7**	**92.4**	**92.3**	**91.6**	**90.6**	**91.5**	**79.2**
Local Range	**90.3 - 100.0**	**87.2 - 100.0**	**84.7 - 98.2**	**87.4 - 98.2**	**80.8 - 97.5**	**71.6 - 100.0**	**52.2 - 91.0**

* Including on the outside of the school building, on playing fields, or other areas of the campus.
† Used to transport students.
‡ Prohibited students from wearing tobacco brand-name apparel or carrying merchandise with tobacco company names, logos, or cartoon characters.
§ In school buildings, on school grounds, on school buses or other vehicles, in school publications, and through sponsorship of school events; and prohibiting students from wearing tobacco brand name apparel or carrying merchandise with tobacco company names, logos, or cartoon characters.
|| Survey did not include schools from the New York City Department of Education.

TABLE 34. Percentage of All Schools That Provided Referrals to Tobacco Cessation Programs for Specific Groups and Posted Signs Marking a Tobacco-Free School Zone,* Selected U.S. Sites: School Health Profiles, Principal Surveys, 2006

	Provided Referrals		
Site	Faculty and Staff	Students	Posted signs marking a tobacco-free school zone
STATE SURVEYS			
Alabama	13.2	19.7	77.9
Alaska	11.8	36.4	68.4
Arizona	21.9	41.0	83.4
Arkansas	15.7	33.0	85.2
Connecticut	24.6	48.3	38.0
Delaware	29.8	55.8	70.9
Florida	23.4	49.8	61.3
Georgia	23.1	24.0	64.7
Hawaii	17.9	61.9	66.5
Idaho	17.4	65.2	62.3
Illinois	16.8	35.4	55.7
Iowa	17.5	47.5	59.8
Kansas	12.0	32.7	56.3
Maine	38.3	67.6	72.5
Massachusetts	36.9	53.2	61.4
Michigan	16.6	45.6	56.3
Mississippi	10.5	17.8	85.3
Missouri	14.0	24.4	56.4
Montana	13.2	44.0	93.2
Nebraska	20.5	40.4	60.9
New Hampshire	40.4	63.5	83.0
New York†	32.1	56.7	72.6
North Carolina	29.9	50.2	74.0
North Dakota	28.9	44.2	71.1
Oregon	29.3	63.2	79.1
Pennsylvania	22.1	62.3	62.0
Rhode Island	39.0	70.8	73.2
South Carolina	25.4	39.0	47.1
South Dakota	11.6	30.5	59.5
Tennessee	9.9	33.5	59.6
Texas	11.1	23.9	80.7
Utah	21.4	81.2	54.7
Vermont	32.1	65.8	68.9
Virginia	22.5	50.8	61.2
Washington	29.0	74.3	88.4
West Virginia	35.8	71.4	90.7
State Median	**22.0**	**47.9**	**67.5**
State Range	**9.9 - 40.4**	**17.8 - 81.2**	**38.0 - 93.2**

TABLE 34. Percentage of All Schools That Provided Referrals to Tobacco Cessation Programs for Specific Groups and Posted Signs Marking a Tobacco-Free School Zone,* Selected U.S. Sites: School Health Profiles, Principal Surveys, 2006 *(continued)*

	Provided Referrals		
Site	Faculty and Staff	Students	Posted signs marking a tobacco-free school zone
LOCAL SURVEYS			
Charlotte-Mecklenburg County	24.3	83.1	88.2
Chicago	12.3	19.8	41.3
Dallas	12.4	30.6	81.7
District of Columbia	16.5	39.2	66.9
Hillsborough County	11.3	49.8	47.4
Los Angeles	39.5	85.9	85.3
Memphis	20.4	60.3	54.7
Miami	27.3	44.9	83.3
Orange County	32.9	57.1	85.1
Philadelphia	15.4	38.3	28.4
San Diego	42.7	96.4	79.5
San Francisco	21.0	77.3	82.5
Local Median	**20.7**	**53.5**	**80.6**
Local Range	**11.3 - 42.7**	**19.8 - 96.4**	**28.4 - 88.2**

* Prohibited the use of all tobacco, including cigarettes, smokeless tobacco (i.e., chewing tobacco, snuff, or dip), cigars, and pipes; by students, faculty and school staff, and visitors; in school buildings, outside on school grounds (including parking lots and playing fields), on school buses or other vehicles used to transport students, and at off-campus school-sponsored events.

† Survey did not include schools from the New York City Department of Education.

TABLE 35a. Percentage of All Schools That Implemented Specific Safety and Security Measures, Selected U.S. Sites: School Health Profiles, Principal Surveys, 2006

Site	Required visitors to report to main office or reception area upon arrival	Maintained a closed campus	Used staff or adult volunteers to monitor halls during and between classes	Routinely conducted locker searches	Required school uniforms
STATE SURVEYS					
Alabama	100.0	97.5	96.5	66.6	21.7
Alaska	92.3	40.8	74.2	25.0	2.8
Arizona	99.7	86.7	90.2	20.1	30.2
Arkansas	100.0	97.1	91.6	61.8	8.6
Connecticut	99.5	94.7	84.4	17.5	7.6
Delaware	100.0	95.5	94.0	29.9	22.6
Florida	100.0	91.5	95.3	40.0	26.6
Georgia	100.0	96.8	96.0	62.2	4.6
Hawaii	98.4	94.1	88.5	2.3	32.2
Idaho	98.4	54.0	94.5	62.2	0.0
Illinois	100.0	86.1	84.1	56.6	4.9
Iowa	98.4	75.6	87.5	40.1	0.7
Kansas	99.2	84.5	93.7	45.0	1.7
Maine	97.7	83.3	74.3	20.8	0.3
Massachusetts	99.6	90.1	85.2	30.9	6.5
Michigan	99.4	88.1	87.5	53.9	14.6
Mississippi	100.0	94.9	93.8	58.9	24.9
Missouri	100.0	95.9	88.9	56.1	4.4
Montana	99.2	43.6	91.9	55.4	0.4
Nebraska	99.1	71.7	92.5	52.6	0.4
New Hampshire	99.5	82.3	81.5	16.7	0.0
New York*	99.8	83.2	87.2	42.6	2.6
North Carolina	100.0	90.4	92.9	56.3	9.1
North Dakota	95.0	52.9	90.9	42.1	1.3
Oregon	99.1	66.4	87.8	33.1	0.9
Pennsylvania	100.0	91.2	89.6	47.8	21.9
Rhode Island	98.8	93.2	89.7	33.7	2.3
South Carolina	100.0	93.9	93.0	60.2	6.8
South Dakota	95.8	59.5	91.3	56.3	0.0
Tennessee	100.0	98.4	92.3	62.1	13.9
Texas	100.0	85.5	95.9	60.7	20.0
Utah	98.3	58.9	91.4	56.9	3.3
Vermont	100.0	75.2	73.9	12.4	0.7
Virginia	100.0	95.7	93.3	49.4	3.2
Washington	99.7	72.0	87.8	26.6	3.5
West Virginia	100.0	97.9	92.2	66.5	0.4
State Median	**99.7**	**87.4**	**91.1**	**48.6**	**4.0**
State Range	**92.3 - 100.0**	**40.8 - 98.4**	**73.9 - 96.5**	**2.3 - 66.6**	**0.0 - 32.2**

TABLE 35a. Percentage of All Schools That Implemented Specific Safety and Security Measures, Selected U.S. Sites: School Health Profiles, Principal Surveys, 2006 *(continued)*

Site	Required visitors to report to main office or reception area upon arrival	Maintained a closed campus	Used staff or adult volunteers to monitor halls during and between classes	Routinely conducted locker searches	Required school uniforms
LOCAL SURVEYS					
Charlotte-Mecklenburg County	100.0	95.1	97.7	57.1	14.2
Chicago	100.0	97.0	92.3	40.2	77.6
Dallas	100.0	93.7	95.8	50.1	68.7
District of Columbia	100.0	93.2	87.4	67.8	34.6
Hillsborough County	100.0	100.0	94.6	35.1	22.6
Los Angeles	98.9	96.7	96.8	62.7	41.6
Memphis	100.0	100.0	96.7	71.3	100.0
Miami	100.0	97.7	94.5	22.2	69.0
Orange County	100.0	100.0	96.9	30.4	0.0
Philadelphia	99.0	98.3	93.7	35.9	97.5
San Diego	100.0	100.0	92.8	7.7	14.5
San Francisco	100.0	77.9	91.6	17.8	31.8
Local Median	**100.0**	**97.4**	**94.6**	**38.1**	**38.1**
Local Range	**98.9 - 100.0**	**77.9 - 100.0**	**87.4 - 97.7**	**7.7 - 71.3**	**0.0 - 100.0**

* Survey did not include schools from the New York City Department of Education.

TABLE 35b. Percentage of All Schools That Implemented Specific Safety and Security Measures, Selected U.S. Sites: School Health Profiles, Principal Surveys, 2006

Site	Required students to wear identification badges	Used metal detectors	Used security or surveillance cameras	Used police, school resource officers, or security guards during the regular school day
STATE SURVEYS				
Alabama	10.7	37.6	85.2	65.7
Alaska	1.3	1.9	20.5	20.2
Arizona	13.5	3.6	30.2	50.2
Arkansas	9.0	17.7	55.5	63.9
Connecticut	8.3	4.8	49.0	57.8
Delaware	3.0	3.0	65.6	67.0
Florida	18.4	22.2	55.5	85.1
Georgia	13.3	29.7	75.5	85.5
Hawaii	42.8	1.6	20.9	76.9
Idaho	2.6	0.9	58.2	64.0
Illinois	10.7	6.2	58.2	38.2
Iowa	1.5	0.8	35.0	24.1
Kansas	4.4	3.1	40.2	41.3
Maine	1.0	1.4	35.1	28.6
Massachusetts	12.4	6.9	55.6	53.6
Michigan	11.3	10.8	54.4	47.8
Mississippi	12.2	30.7	69.9	67.6
Missouri	10.4	7.7	50.9	51.2
Montana	1.7	2.4	35.5	35.4
Nebraska	1.3	1.2	42.7	26.1
New Hampshire	4.3	1.1	34.2	48.1
New York*	9.1	6.8	64.3	64.5
North Carolina	6.1	27.0	64.4	81.6
North Dakota	1.9	2.6	30.9	14.9
Oregon	1.6	0.0	36.5	43.8
Pennsylvania	9.5	19.8	74.6	53.9
Rhode Island	4.5	0.0	46.0	61.2
South Carolina	40.8	29.0	68.0	90.1
South Dakota	3.8	1.4	65.2	24.8
Tennessee	10.8	26.4	85.3	68.0
Texas	21.0	17.3	56.2	61.5
Utah	2.8	0.0	67.0	70.9
Vermont	0.7	0.8	30.1	30.5
Virginia	6.5	25.3	63.2	89.0
Washington	3.4	3.3	44.0	52.7
West Virginia	4.6	12.2	69.3	32.9
State Median	**6.3**	**4.2**	**55.5**	**53.8**
State Range	**0.7 - 42.8**	**0.0 - 37.6**	**20.5 - 85.3**	**14.9 - 90.1**

TABLE 35b. Percentage of All Schools That Implemented Specific Safety and Security Measures, Selected U.S. Sites: School Health Profiles, Principal Surveys, 2006 *(continued)*

Site	Required students to wear identification badges	Used metal detectors	Used security or surveillance cameras	Used police, school resource officers, or security guards during the regular school day
LOCAL SURVEYS				
Charlotte-Mecklenburg County	9.6	55.0	39.1	97.7
Chicago	23.3	82.5	79.5	97.9
Dallas	98.0	89.7	31.5	94.0
District of Columbia	66.3	93.2	100.0	100.0
Hillsborough County	17.1	7.6	6.2	100.0
Los Angeles	13.3	95.3	35.4	97.3
Memphis	22.4	95.0	96.6	85.6
Miami	45.2	50.3	74.9	97.7
Orange County	26.7	8.1	90.7	96.9
Philadelphia	34.0	55.2	67.7	100.0
San Diego	19.9	1.8	18.3	81.8
San Francisco	3.2	3.2	33.8	88.5
Local Median	**22.9**	**55.1**	**53.4**	**97.5**
Local Range	**3.2 - 98.0**	**1.8 - 95.3**	**6.2 - 100.0**	**81.8 - 100.0**

* Survey did not include schools from the New York City Department of Education.

TABLE 36. Percentage of All Schools That Had or Participated in Specific Violence Prevention Programs and That Had a Comprehensive Plan to Address Crisis Preparedness, Response, and Recovery in the Event of a Natural Disaster or Other Emergency or Crisis Situation, Selected U.S. Sites: School Health Profiles, Principal Surveys, 2006

	Violence prevention programs				
Site	Peer mediation program	Safe-passage to school program	Program to prevent gang violence	Program to prevent bullying	Comprehensive plan to address crisis preparedness, response, and recovery
STATE SURVEYS					
Alabama	38.3	10.5	36.5	68.3	99.7
Alaska	23.6	3.0	12.8	55.7	96.6
Arizona	39.0	10.4	41.0	68.6	91.0
Arkansas	29.1	5.6	26.6	69.1	99.3
Connecticut	61.4	5.6	21.6	72.0	96.1
Delaware	38.8	6.1	23.8	56.8	100.0
Florida	66.0	14.5	49.4	69.0	99.0
Georgia	60.9	9.1	41.6	66.5	98.8
Hawaii	56.4	3.4	42.0	61.9	98.4
Idaho	43.9	4.2	28.1	59.3	94.9
Illinois	40.9	5.5	25.6	63.7	98.3
Iowa	27.6	2.8	11.5	62.4	97.2
Kansas	23.9	4.0	14.8	58.0	97.9
Maine	32.0	5.1	8.1	65.3	97.1
Massachusetts	57.4	6.0	21.9	67.6	96.4
Michigan	46.5	6.0	18.8	59.6	97.5
Mississippi	21.8	8.1	21.1	30.8	97.6
Missouri	39.1	6.2	18.6	56.7	98.2
Montana	27.2	5.3	19.1	64.9	93.7
Nebraska	19.4	4.9	17.1	61.2	98.7
New Hampshire	48.6	2.2	11.1	69.4	96.5
New York*	57.3	8.0	22.2	69.1	100.0
North Carolina	48.9	8.5	36.3	67.7	99.3
North Dakota	15.8	1.9	16.1	61.7	87.1
Oregon	38.6	4.4	26.0	63.2	95.6
Pennsylvania	54.9	12.5	19.1	72.2	98.5
Rhode Island	47.5	3.5	24.0	55.8	94.1
South Carolina	43.3	8.1	37.6	54.7	98.8
South Dakota	15.8	2.5	8.5	46.5	90.3
Tennessee	42.2	8.8	33.8	76.2	97.2
Texas	37.9	11.1	38.4	64.8	97.6
Utah	40.4	20.8	55.7	72.8	98.5
Vermont	30.8	1.5	8.0	79.6	97.1
Virginia	59.3	8.9	44.9	71.1	100.0
Washington	32.0	5.0	23.9	70.6	98.7
West Virginia	78.8	7.5	27.2	83.6	96.1
State Median	**39.8**	**5.8**	**23.9**	**65.1**	**97.6**
State Range	**15.8 – 78.8**	**1.5 – 20.8**	**8.0 – 55.7**	**30.8 – 83.6**	**87.1 – 100.0**

TABLE 36. Percentage of All Schools That Had or Participated in Specific Violence Prevention Programs and That Had a Comprehensive Plan to Address Crisis Preparedness, Response, and Recovery in the Event of a Natural Disaster or Other Emergency or Crisis Situation, Selected U.S. Sites: School Health Profiles, Principal Surveys, 2006 *(continued)*

	Violence prevention programs				
Site	Peer mediation program	Safe-passage to school program	Program to prevent gang violence	Program to prevent bullying	Comprehensive plan to address crisis preparedness, response, and recovery
LOCAL SURVEYS					
Charlotte-Mecklenburg County	76.3	22.7	53.9	68.1	100.0
Chicago	42.1	60.0	67.4	66.7	98.2
Dallas	64.8	20.7	52.0	53.9	96.0
District of Columbia	80.6	33.7	68.0	45.3	100.0
Hillsborough County	92.5	12.6	55.1	79.6	100.0
Los Angeles	61.1	50.2	60.3	72.8	98.9
Memphis	73.6	12.0	89.7	89.9	100.0
Miami	88.6	27.0	72.3	87.3	100.0
Orange County	93.8	41.6	84.5	96.9	100.0
Philadelphia	66.4	39.9	50.8	78.6	99.0
San Diego	42.0	7.1	42.1	56.6	100.0
San Francisco	58.1	6.5	55.9	78.3	100.0
Local Median	**70.0**	**24.9**	**58.1**	**75.6**	**100.0**
Local Range	**42.0 - 93.8**	**6.5 - 60.0**	**42.1 - 89.7**	**45.3 - 96.9**	**96.0 - 100.0**

* Survey did not include schools from the New York City Department of Education.

TABLE 37. Percentage of All Schools That Had a School Nurse Who Provided Standard Health Services and the Percentage Where a Student Would Ever Be Permitted to Carry and Self-Administer Specific Medications, Selected U.S. Sites: School Health Profiles, Principal Surveys, 2006

		Medication				
Site	School nurse who provided standard health services to students	Prescription quick-relief inhaler	Epinephrine auto-injector (e.g., EpiPen®)	Insulin or other injected medications	Any other prescribed medications	Any over-the-counter medications
STATE SURVEYS						
Alabama	93.3	72.6	35.6	20.9	2.6	3.1
Alaska	38.1	67.3	36.3	31.5	21.2	27.3
Arizona	66.7	62.1	34.2	20.0	5.8	7.8
Arkansas	98.8	82.1	47.1	31.0	7.9	10.5
Connecticut	98.5	66.4	52.5	33.3	9.7	8.9
Delaware	100.0	51.4	23.9	10.5	3.0	4.4
Florida	71.4	65.7	47.4	19.3	6.5	8.4
Georgia	86.7	76.1	36.3	23.1	5.6	8.5
Hawaii	74.0	80.5	44.7	31.0	43.1	49.0
Idaho	63.1	86.7	55.4	52.7	29.1	39.8
Illinois	78.7	78.6	43.6	25.4	7.3	9.1
Iowa	85.9	80.7	45.1	27.4	12.1	24.7
Kansas	82.8	84.5	49.7	40.0	16.6	25.5
Maine	92.6	82.5	58.9	33.4	5.6	9.3
Massachusetts	98.8	66.7	52.6	23.9	6.7	9.9
Michigan	32.2	85.5	48.3	33.3	15.6	14.3
Mississippi	71.6	69.4	32.3	29.0	13.2	13.2
Missouri	98.2	67.8	29.9	21.6	8.7	14.4
Montana	59.3	87.6	45.5	46.8	21.7	33.8
Nebraska	87.3	75.9	29.6	32.3	11.4	19.7
New Hampshire	98.9	78.3	64.1	35.4	3.9	6.0
New York*	99.3	62.1	44.0	27.6	11.6	14.8
North Carolina	91.9	87.1	55.7	44.1	18.1	20.3
North Dakota	28.9	86.6	51.0	49.5	23.8	30.5
Oregon	60.9	68.6	35.5	29.9	15.4	30.7
Pennsylvania	99.7	71.4	42.1	18.8	3.3	5.2
Rhode Island	98.8	72.2	58.1	36.0	11.8	21.0
South Carolina	97.2	75.7	48.0	34.9	14.0	11.1
South Dakota	59.4	79.5	33.6	34.7	25.2	42.2
Tennessee	89.3	73.4	43.3	25.6	4.6	6.0
Texas	95.0	76.1	40.1	28.4	5.3	5.6
Utah	71.7	95.1	63.8	64.4	45.2	59.3
Vermont	99.3	69.0	53.6	43.1	10.7	13.8
Virginia	96.7	78.0	51.7	22.3	5.7	8.5
Washington	92.9	81.7	47.5	36.6	15.9	20.7
West Virginia	95.5	68.8	32.3	25.8	8.5	11.4
State Median	**90.6**	**76.0**	**45.3**	**31.0**	**11.1**	**13.5**
State Range	**28.9 - 100.0**	**51.4 - 95.1**	**23.9 - 64.1**	**10.5 - 64.4**	**2.6 - 45.2**	**3.1 - 59.3**

TABLE 37. Percentage of All Schools That Had a School Nurse Who Provided Standard Health Services and the Percentage Where a Student Would Ever Be Permitted to Carry and Self-Administer Specific Medications, Selected U.S. Sites: School Health Profiles, Principal Surveys, 2006 *(continued)*

		Medication				
Site	School nurse who provided standard health services to students	Prescription quick-relief inhaler	Epinephrine auto-injector (e.g., EpiPen®)	Insulin or other injected medications	Any other prescribed medications	Any over-the-counter medications
LOCAL SURVEYS						
Charlotte-Mecklenburg County	97.7	73.3	62.6	36.7	14.7	9.8
Chicago	91.0	73.6	26.5	21.8	19.8	10.6
Dallas	98.0	43.2	8.3	2.1	2.1	8.3
District of Columbia	100.0	63.3	14.7	4.0	10.8	13.7
Hillsborough County	97.9	64.5	36.9	10.8	1.7	7.3
Los Angeles	98.9	46.3	23.7	14.9	12.7	13.9
Memphis	96.6	69.0	27.6	24.1	22.3	20.3
Miami	16.0	75.6	67.7	41.6	22.8	31.4
Orange County	83.9	67.1	36.0	11.8	2.5	2.5
Philadelphia	100.0	48.8	13.0	7.2	6.2	8.5
San Diego	98.3	66.4	33.7	36.2	22.9	22.9
San Francisco	31.0	79.5	35.7	30.3	34.3	31.1
Local Median	**97.8**	**66.8**	**30.7**	**18.4**	**13.7**	**12.2**
Local Range	**16.0 - 100.0**	**43.2 - 79.5**	**8.3 - 67.7**	**2.1 - 41.6**	**1.7 - 34.3**	**2.5 - 31.4**

* Survey did not include schools from the New York City Department of Education.

TABLE 38. Percentage of All Schools That Provided Specific Health Services to Students, Selected U.S. Sites: School Health Profiles, Principal Surveys, 2006

Site	Identification or school-based management of chronic health conditions	Identification or school-based management of acute illnesses	Asthma Action Plan or Individualized Health Plan for all students with asthma	Immunizations	Assistance with enrolling in Medicaid or SCHIP*
STATE SURVEYS					
Alabama	82.8	73.4	80.9	45.8	59.9
Alaska	52.5	43.3	34.0	67.4	42.0
Arizona	70.7	60.2	50.1	51.4	47.1
Arkansas	72.5	66.1	67.0	48.5	58.9
Connecticut	80.3	73.5	76.4	41.5	48.8
Delaware	95.5	87.8	75.8	61.2	53.8
Florida	74.2	67.7	65.1	54.5	47.3
Georgia	73.0	63.4	58.3	34.7	37.0
Hawaii	73.8	66.7	75.7	41.4	47.5
Idaho	57.3	50.6	43.5	44.4	53.4
Illinois	69.3	60.3	59.4	41.3	48.0
Iowa	74.6	66.6	58.4	51.4	65.5
Kansas	62.6	55.4	47.9	51.0	55.4
Maine	77.2	69.9	63.0	42.8	49.7
Massachusetts	88.5	82.4	75.1	51.8	73.4
Michigan	54.8	43.4	41.9	39.1	42.0
Mississippi	49.5	43.5	36.0	32.1	44.8
Missouri	79.4	73.4	72.9	60.4	56.2
Montana	61.5	51.9	57.3	61.8	55.3
Nebraska	82.5	69.2	86.8	57.6	58.2
New Hampshire	87.4	79.8	68.5	53.3	75.8
New York†	79.5	73.6	56.7	49.7	51.4
North Carolina	90.4	78.8	82.7	60.1	47.9
North Dakota	51.0	39.0	42.0	80.7	41.4
Oregon	63.2	55.9	55.0	50.1	54.4
Pennsylvania	81.8	74.6	67.7	48.7	66.1
Rhode Island	65.6	59.3	53.6	59.6	51.6
South Carolina	84.5	77.0	67.2	55.3	65.9
South Dakota	38.9	34.3	22.8	44.8	45.8
Tennessee	72.4	63.4	67.5	46.1	37.5
Texas	82.8	74.6	65.6	64.2	62.7
Utah	70.7	64.8	62.6	53.6	51.8
Vermont	92.8	81.4	70.1	49.5	86.4
Virginia	85.4	75.2	75.5	39.4	55.6
Washington	83.9	77.3	81.1	48.2	78.6
West Virginia	86.0	78.0	75.0	44.0	65.4
State Median	**74.4**	**67.2**	**65.4**	**49.9**	**53.6**
State Range	**38.9 - 95.5**	**34.3 - 87.8**	**22.8 - 86.8**	**32.1 - 80.7**	**37.0 - 86.4**

TABLE 38. Percentage of All Schools That Provided Specific Health Services to Students, Selected U.S. Sites: School Health Profiles, Principal Surveys, 2006 *(continued)*

Site	Identification or school-based management of chronic health conditions	Identification or school-based management of acute illnesses	Asthma Action Plan or Individualized Health Plan for all students with asthma	Immunizations	Assistance with enrolling in Medicaid or SCHIP*
LOCAL SURVEYS					
Charlotte-Mecklenburg County	87.8	68.3	80.2	41.6	50.2
Chicago	81.0	70.1	74.7	66.9	71.2
Dallas	73.7	67.7	67.1	59.6	66.7
District of Columbia	89.2	63.0	51.0	76.8	33.3
Hillsborough County	79.3	68.8	64.5	69.3	52.4
Los Angeles	79.4	74.9	71.2	62.2	66.0
Memphis	74.0	65.2	71.3	48.0	44.6
Miami	38.8	32.9	19.7	47.5	38.3
Orange County	70.8	66.9	64.6	65.8	67.7
Philadelphia	92.8	87.8	86.9	51.5	85.8
San Diego	94.5	85.5	79.7	69.5	83.8
San Francisco	71.0	65.0	49.3	36.1	29.4
Local Median	**79.4**	**68.0**	**69.2**	**60.9**	**59.2**
Local Range	**38.8 - 94.5**	**32.9 - 87.8**	**19.7 - 86.9**	**36.1 - 76.8**	**29.4 - 85.8**

* State Children's Health Insurance Program.
† Survey did not include schools from the New York City Department of Education.

TABLE 39a. Percentage of All Schools with a Policy on Students and/or Staff who Have HIV* Infection or AIDS† and Among Those Schools, Percentage Whose Policy Addressed Specific Issues, Selected U.S. Sites: School Health Profiles, Principal Surveys, 2006

		Issue addressed by policy			
Site	Had a policy	Attendance at school of students with HIV infection	Procedures to protect HIV-infected students and staff from discrimination	Maintenance of confidentiality of HIV-infected students and staff	Work site safety
STATE SURVEYS					
Alabama	62.2	96.5	98.5	99.3	100.0
Alaska	40.5	90.5	94.7	93.5	93.6
Arizona	41.7	91.9	96.3	96.2	98.4
Arkansas	33.1	90.6	98.9	98.6	98.2
Connecticut	59.3	92.3	97.7	98.5	96.2
Delaware	30.3	100.0	100.0	100.0	94.8
Florida	43.9	90.6	96.7	100.0	100.0
Georgia	42.6	92.1	99.2	100.0	99.1
Hawaii	51.2	93.0	100.0	100.0	100.0
Idaho	60.4	93.0	93.3	96.0	94.0
Illinois	39.7	92.2	96.2	99.2	99.2
Iowa	42.9	95.1	94.1	95.0	96.6
Kansas	39.6	94.9	95.0	100.0	98.0
Maine	66.4	96.7	97.9	99.5	99.4
Massachusetts	58.2	93.3	97.8	98.9	97.0
Michigan	32.3	90.1	95.5	98.3	100.0
Mississippi	27.0	97.6	95.1	92.7	97.6
Missouri	52.9	91.5	96.0	98.1	96.7
Montana	48.3	94.4	97.8	99.3	94.7
Nebraska	53.5	94.2	95.9	99.2	96.9
New Hampshire	76.9	94.5	99.3	100.0	98.4
New York‡	59.0	85.2	96.5	99.0	97.5
North Carolina	36.0	91.1	95.7	99.0	100.0
North Dakota	39.7	93.6	96.8	98.5	96.8
Oregon	66.4	94.9	98.4	99.0	98.9
Pennsylvania	59.9	92.8	98.1	99.6	98.0
Rhode Island	64.8	98.2	100.0	100.0	100.0
South Carolina	57.9	92.7	96.5	100.0	99.3
South Dakota	51.9	95.8	95.1	98.0	95.6
Tennessee	58.2	93.6	98.8	99.4	98.2
Texas	30.8	87.7	95.4	98.9	95.9
Utah	52.5	98.2	99.1	99.1	100.0
Vermont	89.5	97.6	99.2	100.0	100.0
Virginia	55.2	90.2	96.6	98.6	96.5
Washington	45.4	94.8	97.9	97.9	98.9
West Virginia	27.1	93.8	100.0	100.0	97.9
State Median	**51.6**	**93.5**	**97.3**	**99.1**	**98.1**
State Range	**27.0 – 89.5**	**85.2 – 100.0**	**93.3 – 100.0**	**92.7 – 100.0**	**93.6 – 100.0**

TABLE 39a. Percentage of All Schools with a Policy on Students and/or Staff who Have HIV* Infection or AIDS† and Among Those Schools, Percentage Whose Policy Addressed Specific Issues, Selected U.S. Sites: School Health Profiles, Principal Surveys, 2006 *(continued)*

		Issue addressed by policy			
Site	Had a policy	Attendance at school of students with HIV infection	Procedures to protect HIV-infected students and staff from discrimination	Maintenance of confidentiality of HIV-infected students and staff	Work site safety
LOCAL SURVEYS					
Charlotte-Mecklenburg County	35.2	93.0	93.0	93.0	93.0
Chicago	48.3	90.4	100.0	100.0	99.0
Dallas	30.5	93.0	100.0	100.0	100.0
District of Columbia	28.1	65.4	100.0	100.0	75.7
Hillsborough County	45.3	82.8	100.0	100.0	100.0
Los Angeles	57.7	91.5	98.0	100.0	97.5
Memphis	51.1	89.8	100.0	100.0	100.0
Miami	44.6	78.3	97.3	100.0	91.8
Orange County	37.8	100.0	100.0	100.0	100.0
Philadelphia	57.7	85.2	100.0	100.0	100.0
San Diego	100.0	97.6	100.0	100.0	100.0
San Francisco	50.0	100.0	100.0	100.0	100.0
Local Median	**46.8**	**91.0**	**100.0**	**100.0**	**100.0**
Local Range	**28.1 - 100.0**	**65.4 - 100.0**	**93.0 - 100.0**	**93.0 - 100.0**	**75.7 - 100.0**

* Human immunodeficiency virus.
† Acquired immunodeficiency syndrome.
‡ Survey did not include schools from the New York City Department of Education.

TABLE 39b. Percentage of All Schools with a Policy on Students and/or Staff who Have HIV* Infection or AIDS† and Among Those Schools, Percentage Whose Policy Addressed Specific Issues, Selected U.S. Sites: School Health Profiles, Principal Surveys, 2006

	Issue addressed by policy			
Site	Confidential counseling for HIV-infected students	Communication of the policy to students, school staff, and parents	Adequate training about HIV infection for school staff	Procedure for implementing the policy
STATE SURVEYS				
Alabama	91.0	95.0	92.3	95.3
Alaska	73.7	84.7	83.7	87.6
Arizona	73.9	83.0	89.3	91.7
Arkansas	88.7	97.4	86.8	96.1
Connecticut	76.2	83.5	87.1	88.2
Delaware	89.4	78.9	89.5	94.8
Florida	87.7	89.1	87.5	94.5
Georgia	82.1	92.0	87.0	90.2
Hawaii	77.6	82.0	91.8	95.7
Idaho	73.9	77.3	67.2	84.7
Illinois	79.2	95.8	94.8	98.0
Iowa	72.7	84.7	90.9	93.1
Kansas	75.6	89.4	87.6	88.6
Maine	78.8	81.7	92.7	91.2
Massachusetts	79.1	84.8	76.0	86.0
Michigan	78.0	85.0	88.1	88.8
Mississippi	85.5	95.3	90.5	95.4
Missouri	76.5	87.9	83.5	93.6
Montana	85.6	93.4	80.2	94.5
Nebraska	75.9	90.1	83.9	92.6
New Hampshire	74.7	85.8	79.6	89.7
New York ‡	68.9	82.9	87.1	86.0
North Carolina	78.5	90.7	91.0	92.9
North Dakota	81.6	95.5	90.8	96.9
Oregon	80.1	89.4	90.4	96.0
Pennsylvania	73.3	89.5	79.7	93.3
Rhode Island	79.9	94.4	94.7	96.3
South Carolina	89.1	86.0	95.5	94.1
South Dakota	83.0	93.8	78.6	87.9
Tennessee	84.7	91.6	85.3	94.0
Texas	85.0	86.2	91.1	94.3
Utah	77.0	86.6	81.5	89.1
Vermont	73.8	86.9	91.8	91.7
Virginia	79.9	83.8	89.2	90.3
Washington	75.5	90.4	95.4	96.3
West Virginia	82.4	92.9	80.9	91.6
State Median	**79.0**	**88.5**	**87.9**	**93.0**
State Range	**68.9 - 91.0**	**77.3 - 97.4**	**67.2 - 95.5**	**84.7 - 98.0**

TABLE 39b. Percentage of All Schools with a Policy on Students and/or Staff who Have HIV* Infection or AIDS† and Among Those Schools, Percentage Whose Policy Addressed Specific Issues, Selected U.S. Sites: School Health Profiles, Principal Surveys, 2006 *(continued)*

	Issue addressed by policy			
Site	Confidential counseling for HIV-infected students	Communication of the policy to students, school staff, and parents	Adequate training about HIV infection for school staff	Procedure for implementing the policy
LOCAL SURVEYS				
Charlotte-Mecklenburg County	69.5	84.6	86.0	78.7
Chicago	90.4	89.7	81.9	93.4
Dallas	86.6	93.2	93.2	86.3
District of Columbia	69.2	79.5	55.1	79.5
Hillsborough County	91.8	91.8	91.8	95.9
Los Angeles	89.0	90.5	91.0	96.0
Memphis	96.2	100.0	96.8	96.8
Miami	89.3	94.7	78.2	88.8
Orange County	91.5	83.0	100.0	91.5
Philadelphia	78.4	78.3	59.2	84.5
San Diego	90.4	92.8	97.7	100.0
San Francisco	88.1	88.1	87.3	100.0
Local Median	**89.2**	**90.1**	**89.2**	**92.5**
Local Range	**69.2 - 96.2**	**78.3 - 100.0**	**55.1 - 100.0**	**78.7 - 100.0**

* Human immunodeficiency virus.
† Acquired immunodeficiency syndrome.
‡ Survey did not include schools from the New York City Department of Education.

TABLE 40. Percentage of All Schools That Had One or More School Health Councils* and Engaged Parents and Families in Specific Health Education Activities During the 2005–2006 School Year, Selected U.S. Sites: School Health Profiles, Principal and Lead Health Education Teacher Surveys, 2006

Site	School health council	Provided families with information on school health education	Met with a parents' organization to discuss school health education	Invited family members to attend health education classes
STATE SURVEYS				
Alabama	44.5	63.3	30.3	37.2
Alaska	48.7	52.8	17.8	31.6
Arizona	35.6	53.5	19.8	25.3
Arkansas	68.7	64.9	23.6	35.5
Connecticut	60.1	71.8	29.6	32.6
Delaware	63.4	80.3	31.7	37.6
Florida	49.4	62.7	26.0	29.6
Georgia	50.9	66.5	27.3	42.8
Hawaii	47.2	66.2	17.3	32.4
Idaho	49.7	58.9	14.5	42.9
Illinois	55.1	NA†	NA	NA
Iowa	59.5	61.8	16.7	22.3
Kansas	60.6	51.0	10.5	25.0
Maine	69.2	70.2	13.7	32.4
Massachusetts	59.0	80.0	32.8	27.2
Michigan	71.0	70.2	32.2	45.6
Mississippi	34.7	58.8	18.4	38.1
Missouri	69.4	69.6	25.0	28.5
Montana	61.1	63.2	13.1	33.2
Nebraska	54.7	63.3	13.4	24.5
New Hampshire	64.7	79.3	18.1	31.0
New York‡	67.4	82.7	32.5	28.2
North Carolina	57.9	66.0	22.1	41.4
North Dakota	54.1	54.3	13.6	29.7
Oregon	52.6	77.6	15.6	39.8
Pennsylvania	70.4	67.5	23.7	28.3
Rhode Island	51.8	71.5	32.5	23.0
South Carolina	56.6	67.4	22.3	45.2
South Dakota	46.7	47.6	13.6	21.0
Tennessee	43.4	59.5	26.1	32.2
Texas	63.0	59.7	23.9	31.4
Utah	45.4	64.4	23.0	41.3
Vermont	73.9	80.5	14.0	41.0
Virginia	49.3	73.8	22.2	37.8
Washington	51.4	NA	NA	NA
West Virginia	49.2	67.0	24.8	32.9
State Median	**54.9**	**66.1**	**22.3**	**32.4**
State Range	**34.7 - 73.9**	**47.6 - 82.7**	**10.5 - 32.8**	**21.0 - 45.6**

TABLE 40. Percentage of All Schools That Had One or More School Health Councils* and Engaged Parents and Families in Specific Health Education Activities During the 2005–2006 School Year, Selected U.S. Sites: School Health Profiles, Principal and Lead Health Education Teacher Surveys, 2006 *(continued)*

Site	School health council	Provided families with information on school health education	Met with a parents' organization to discuss school health education	Invited family members to attend health education classes
LOCAL SURVEYS				
Charlotte-Mecklenburg County	34.5	97.4	24.7	64.2
Chicago	37.9	60.0	37.3	31.9
Dallas	24.1	66.7	24.5	40.8
District of Columbia	49.6	59.9	35.5	59.3
Hillsborough County	35.5	57.2	29.7	18.8
Los Angeles	48.9	80.7	34.7	57.4
Memphis	45.4	82.1	63.3	75.4
Miami	51.0	60.5	18.8	26.3
Orange County	62.7	71.8	22.8	42.7
Philadelphia	53.7	53.7	25.4	27.7
San Diego	47.9	79.7	37.8	56.2
San Francisco	79.0	87.9	53.1	29.0
Local Median	**48.4**	**69.3**	**32.2**	**41.8**
Local Range	**24.1 - 79.0**	**53.7 - 97.4**	**18.8 - 63.3**	**18.8 - 75.4**

* A group, committee, or team that offers guidance on the development of policies or coordinates activities on health topics.
† Data not available.
‡ Survey did not include schools from the New York City Department of Education.

TABLE 41. Percentage of All Schools That Asked Students to Participate in Health-Related Community Activities as Part of a Required Health Education Course During the 2005–2006 School Year, Selected U.S. Sites: School Health Profiles, Lead Health Education Teacher Surveys, 2006

Site	Performed volunteer work*	Participated in or attended a health fair	Gathered information about health services†	Visited a store to compare prices of health products	Identified potential injury sites‡	Identified advertising designed to influence health behaviors§	Advocated for a health-related issue	Completed homework or projects that involved family members
STATE SURVEYS								
Alabama	21.4	24.2	47.2	24.7	56.6	57.2	39.1	59.5
Alaska	14.0	30.1	37.1	16.1	34.7	33.3	42.3	53.8
Arizona	6.2	10.5	20.1	9.7	22.4	28.2	23.1	34.1
Arkansas	11.1	19.6	49.4	30.7	59.5	69.4	42.8	72.0
Connecticut	13.4	20.7	33.2	17.3	43.3	61.8	52.3	70.2
Delaware	22.1	32.6	50.3	34.1	61.1	78.4	65.3	75.3
Florida	15.4	14.6	28.2	17.7	30.3	41.5	30.7	44.1
Georgia	17.7	25.8	49.8	28.1	59.5	69.9	44.2	75.1
Hawaii	15.9	28.8	62.3	35.4	54.0	79.5	82.2	77.7
Idaho	16.4	28.4	44.5	30.5	48.6	70.4	49.5	77.9
Iowa	11.1	9.0	29.6	13.1	36.5	46.1	33.4	58.2
Kansas	9.8	12.8	31.9	15.0	30.0	41.4	31.1	59.4
Maine	6.6	11.5	48.8	27.4	48.3	66.0	52.2	72.8
Massachusetts	10.9	16.6	37.0	21.8	40.1	59.8	44.7	68.9
Michigan	9.9	10.1	32.9	15.9	37.7	56.0	38.4	66.2
Mississippi	24.8	30.7	66.4	38.5	70.0	69.0	53.4	77.7
Missouri	10.3	28.1	39.9	22.6	52.3	61.3	41.8	71.2
Montana	10.9	28.9	39.6	21.3	53.1	61.6	45.1	71.0
Nebraska	11.4	16.7	29.2	15.2	43.4	56.1	42.4	68.6
New Hampshire	9.9	16.6	40.2	16.9	43.4	59.9	51.3	71.4
New York‖	23.1	28.5	62.3	31.6	57.5	79.6	71.1	90.2
North Carolina	10.2	24.5	43.5	23.6	51.3	57.7	44.5	71.1
North Dakota	9.8	35.6	42.5	15.2	45.3	61.4	45.9	70.8
Oregon	15.2	18.2	43.5	25.7	51.2	71.5	50.3	78.0
Pennsylvania	17.2	29.1	42.4	25.6	54.9	70.2	48.6	73.5
Rhode Island	18.1	28.0	46.3	28.0	53.3	70.0	63.2	79.6
South Carolina	14.1	20.0	36.0	23.8	48.1	50.9	39.6	59.5
South Dakota	6.7	23.3	21.5	5.6	28.9	33.8	27.7	54.4
Tennessee	12.6	25.0	35.1	18.8	43.6	41.6	32.2	52.1
Texas	13.8	19.1	31.6	23.3	40.5	49.3	33.8	56.5
Utah	15.7	17.1	32.9	26.9	53.5	73.2	47.8	81.8
Vermont	7.6	19.0	29.7	22.1	34.3	64.2	58.1	72.5
Virginia	11.9	16.7	40.0	29.4	48.9	58.0	40.3	67.4
West Virginia	21.9	35.0	57.8	30.1	66.7	77.2	52.0	75.0
State Median	**13.0**	**22.0**	**40.0**	**23.5**	**48.5**	**61.4**	**44.6**	**71.1**
State Range	**6.2 – 24.8**	**9.0 – 35.6**	**20.1 – 66.4**	**5.6 – 38.5**	**22.4 – 70.0**	**28.2 – 79.6**	**23.1 – 82.2**	**34.1 – 90.2**

TABLE 41. Percentage of All Schools That Asked Students to Participate in Health-Related Community Activities as Part of a Required Health Education Course During the 2005–2006 School Year, Selected U.S. Sites: School Health Profiles, Lead Health Education Teacher Surveys, 2006 *(continued)*

Site	Performed volunteer work*	Participated in or attended a health fair	Gathered information about health services†	Visited a store to compare prices of health products	Identified potential injury sites‡	Identified advertising designed to influence health behaviors §	Advocated for a health-related issue	Completed homework or projects that involved family members
LOCAL SURVEYS								
Charlotte-Mecklenburg County	7.9	26.9	37.9	48.8	70.0	75.9	56.5	94.5
Chicago	11.4	16.6	28.7	17.5	32.9	29.5	24.0	44.1
Dallas	16.7	20.8	39.6	22.9	37.5	52.1	33.3	45.8
District of Columbia	20.6	45.4	62.1	38.2	44.8	61.1	58.8	59.1
Hillsborough County	8.1	2.0	24.5	2.0	15.9	31.8	17.9	27.5
Los Angeles	19.5	44.3	62.0	43.0	53.4	88.2	59.7	90.7
Memphis	36.9	55.6	61.0	38.6	65.9	66.3	52.0	74.7
Miami	20.3	20.3	30.4	17.7	30.3	38.4	30.3	43.0
Orange County	13.3	13.6	27.3	21.9	30.0	38.3	38.3	41.2
Philadelphia	19.3	40.4	56.2	34.1	53.0	58.5	49.3	68.3
San Diego¶	0.0	0.0	0.0	0.0	0.0	0.0	0.0	0.0
San Francisco	14.3	40.8	35.7	17.9	28.6	50.0	42.9	50.0
Local Median	**15.5**	**23.9**	**36.8**	**22.4**	**35.2**	**51.1**	**40.6**	**47.9**
Local Range	**0.0 – 36.9**	**0.0 – 55.6**	**0.0 – 62.1**	**0.0 – 48.8**	**0.0 – 70.0**	**0.0 – 88.2**	**0.0 – 59.7**	**0.0 – 94.5**

* At a hospital, a local health department, or any other local organization that addresses health issues.
† That are available in the community.
‡ At school, home, or in the community.
§ In the community.
|| Survey did not include schools from the New York City Department of Education.
¶ San Diego does not have a required health education course, but requires that health education be taught in science and physical education classes.

PROFILES 2006

School Health Profiles Characteristics of Health Programs Among Secondary Schools

Printer:

Please adjust spine width to fit publication

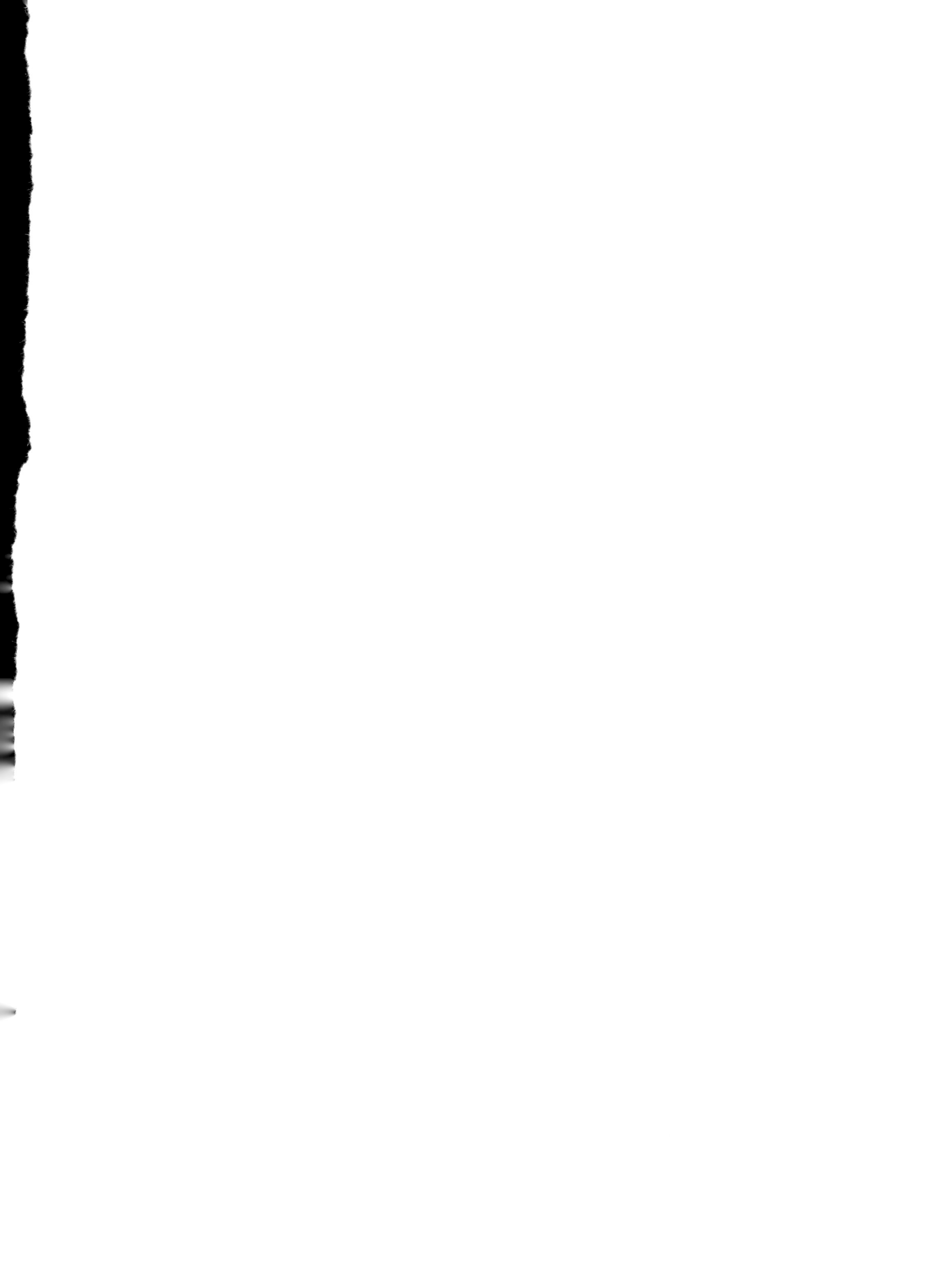

www.ingramcontent.com/pod-product-compliance
Lightning Source LLC
Chambersburg PA
CBHW080246180526
45167CB00006B/2438

* 9 7 8 1 4 9 9 7 0 1 7 0 8 *